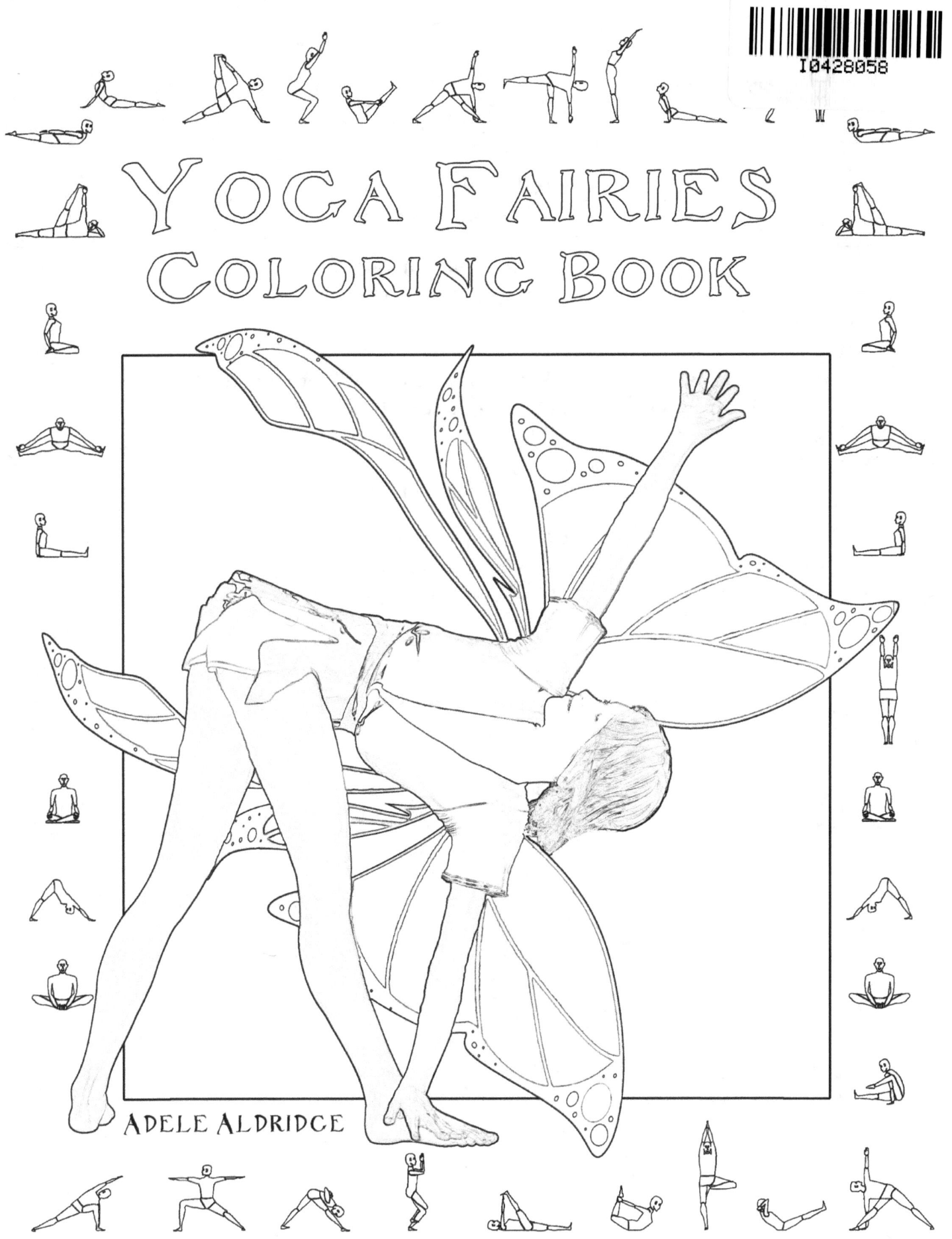

Yoga Fairies
Coloring Book

ADELE ALDRIDGE

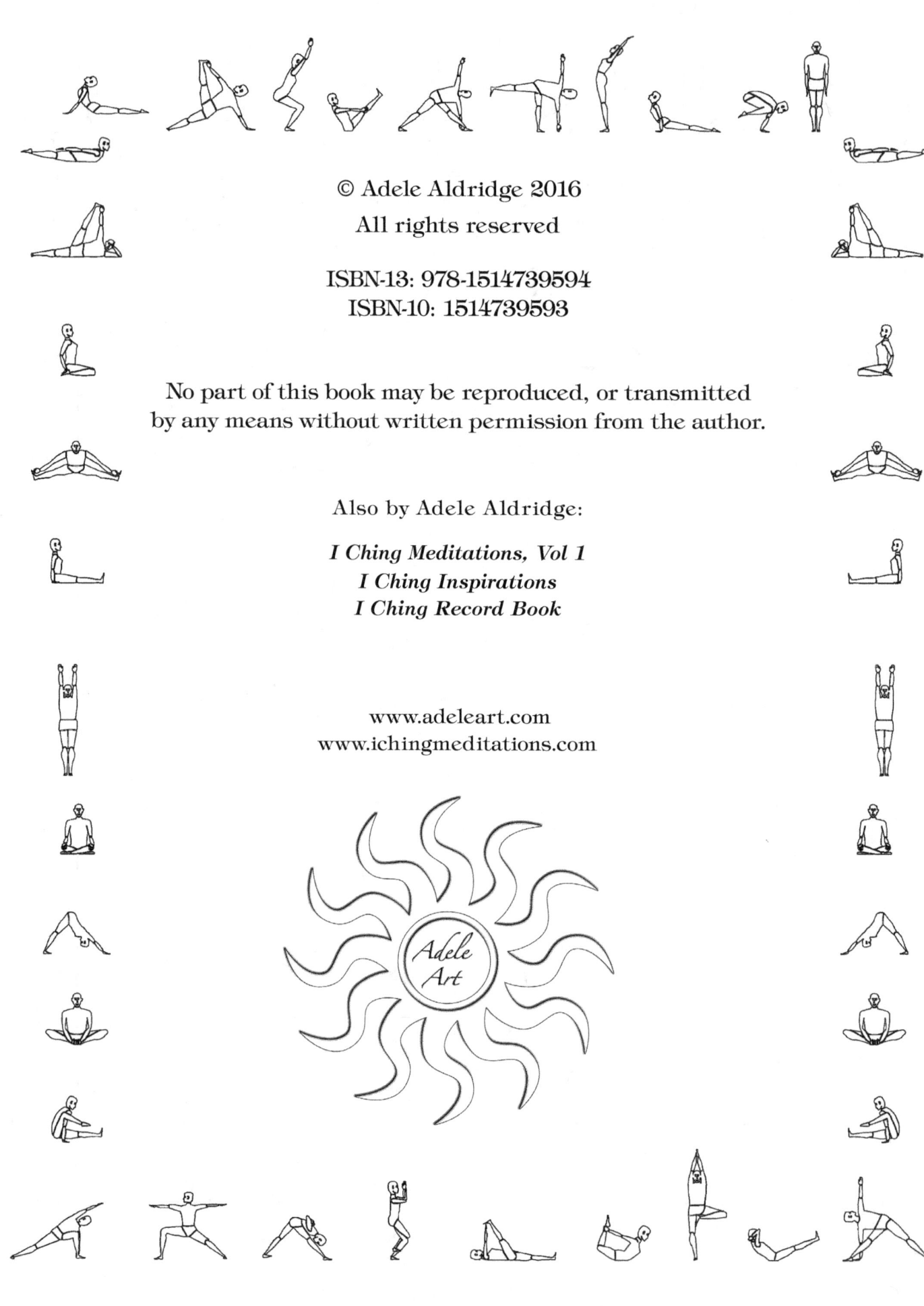

ISBN-13: 978-1514739594
ISBN-10: 1514739593

Also by Adele Aldridge:

I Ching Meditations, Vol 1
I Ching Inspirations
I Ching Record Book

www.adeleart.com
www.ichingmeditations.com

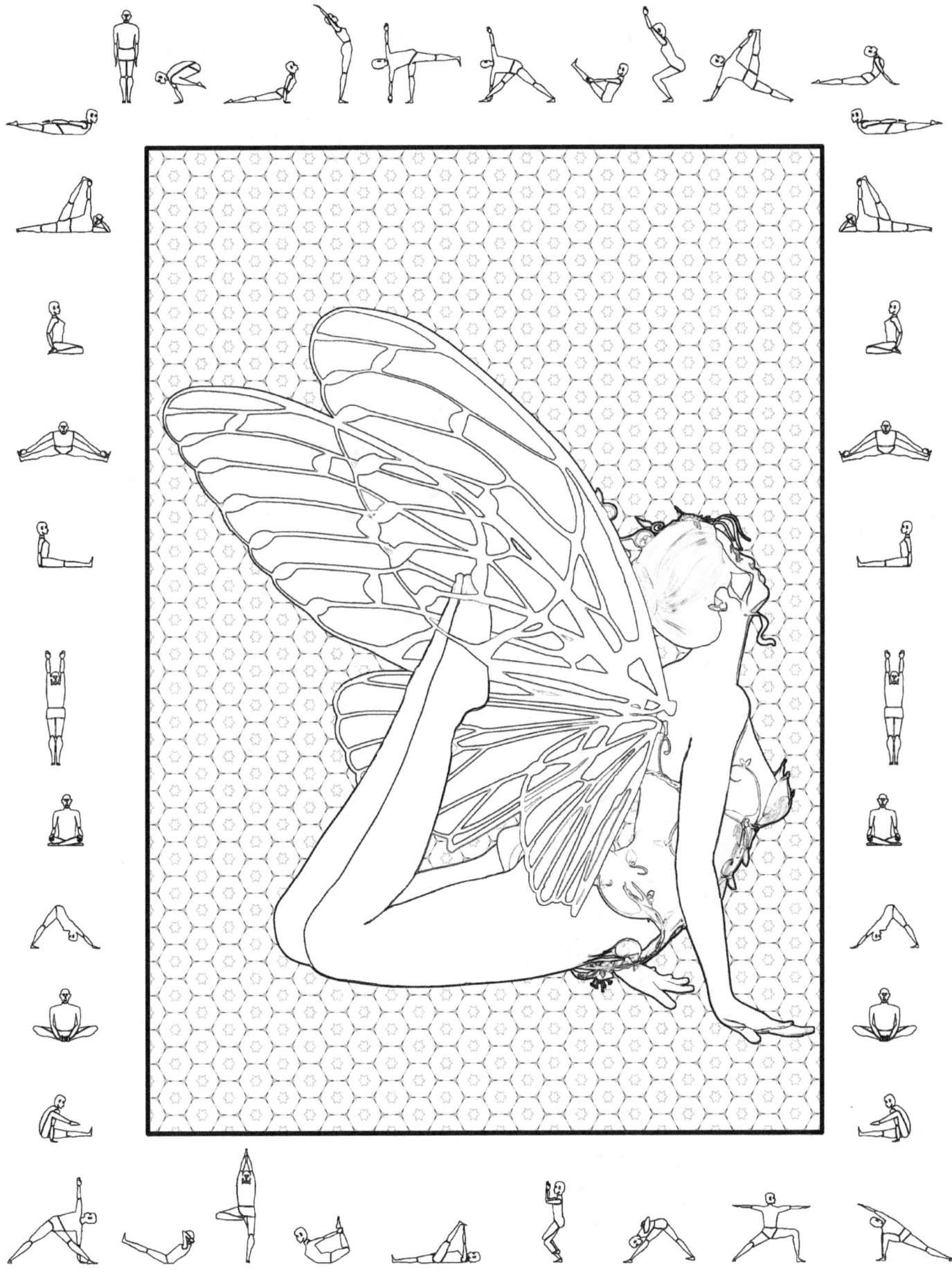

Coloring Yoga Fairies

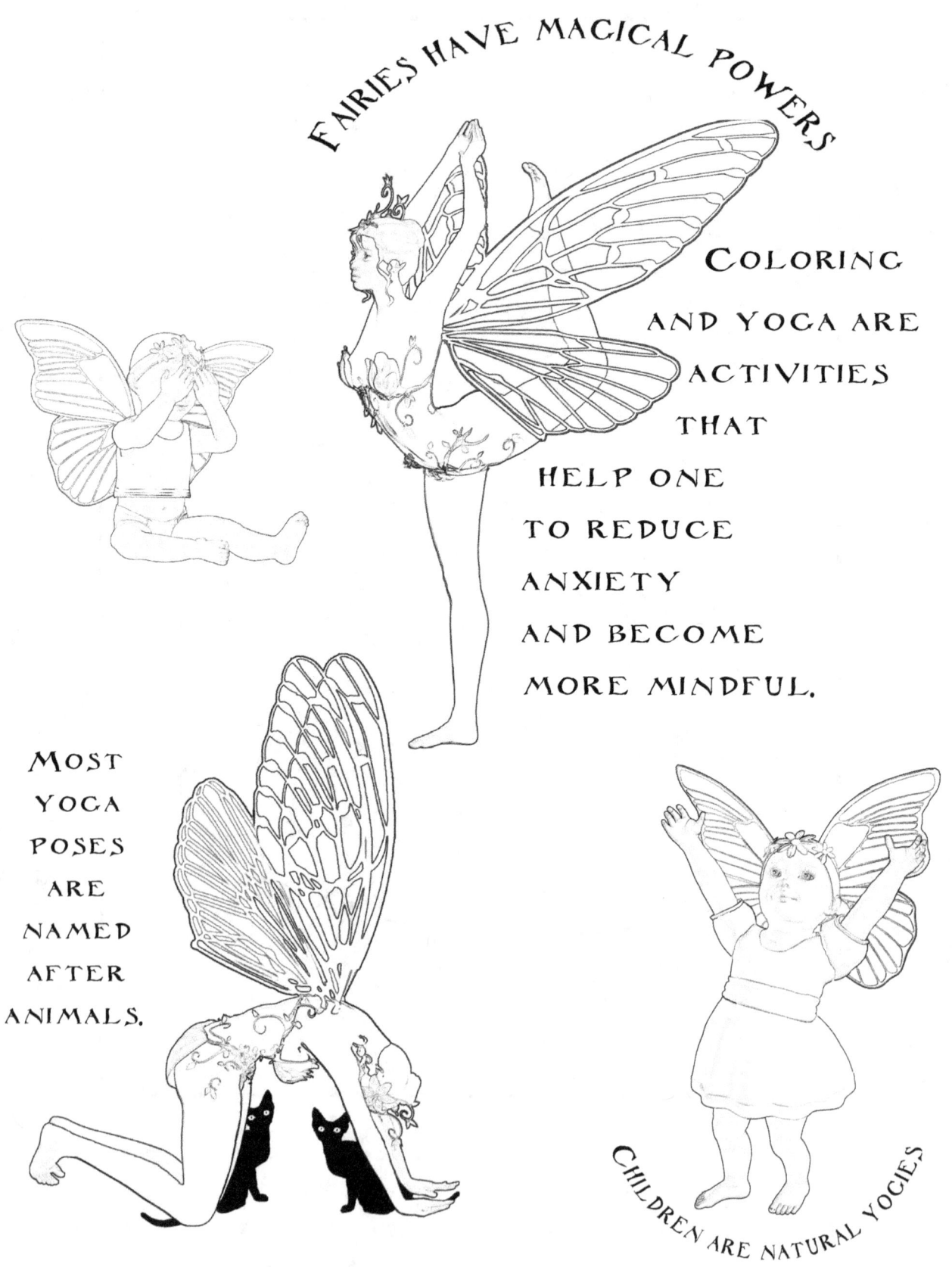

FAIRIES HAVE MAGICAL POWERS

COLORING
AND YOGA ARE
ACTIVITIES
THAT
HELP ONE
TO REDUCE
ANXIETY
AND BECOME
MORE MINDFUL.

MOST
YOGA
POSES
ARE
NAMED
AFTER
ANIMALS.

CHILDREN ARE NATURAL YOGIES

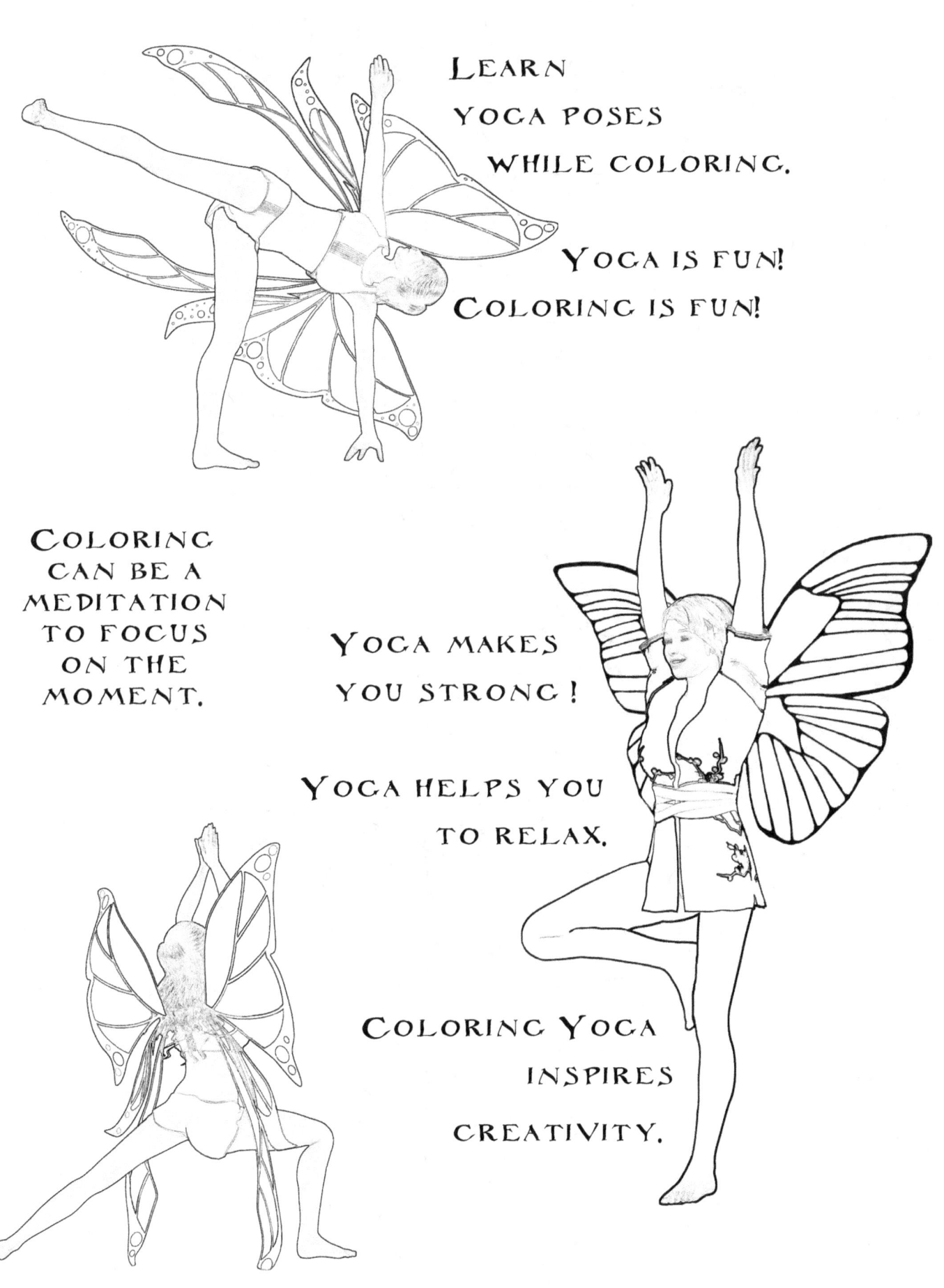

LEARN
YOGA POSES
WHILE COLORING.

YOGA IS FUN!
COLORING IS FUN!

COLORING
CAN BE A
MEDITATION
TO FOCUS
ON THE
MOMENT.

YOGA MAKES
YOU STRONG!

YOGA HELPS YOU
TO RELAX.

COLORING YOGA
INSPIRES
CREATIVITY.

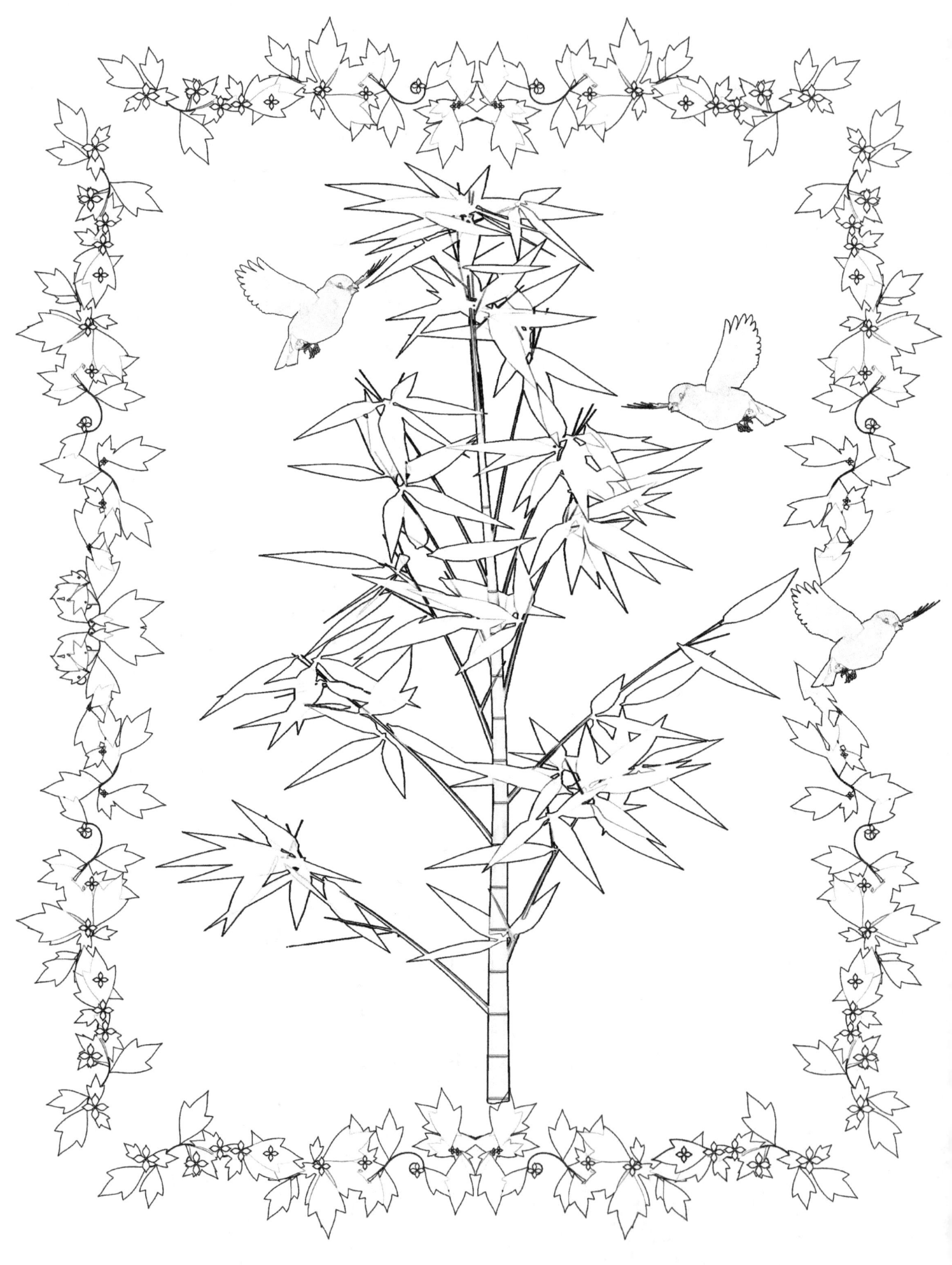

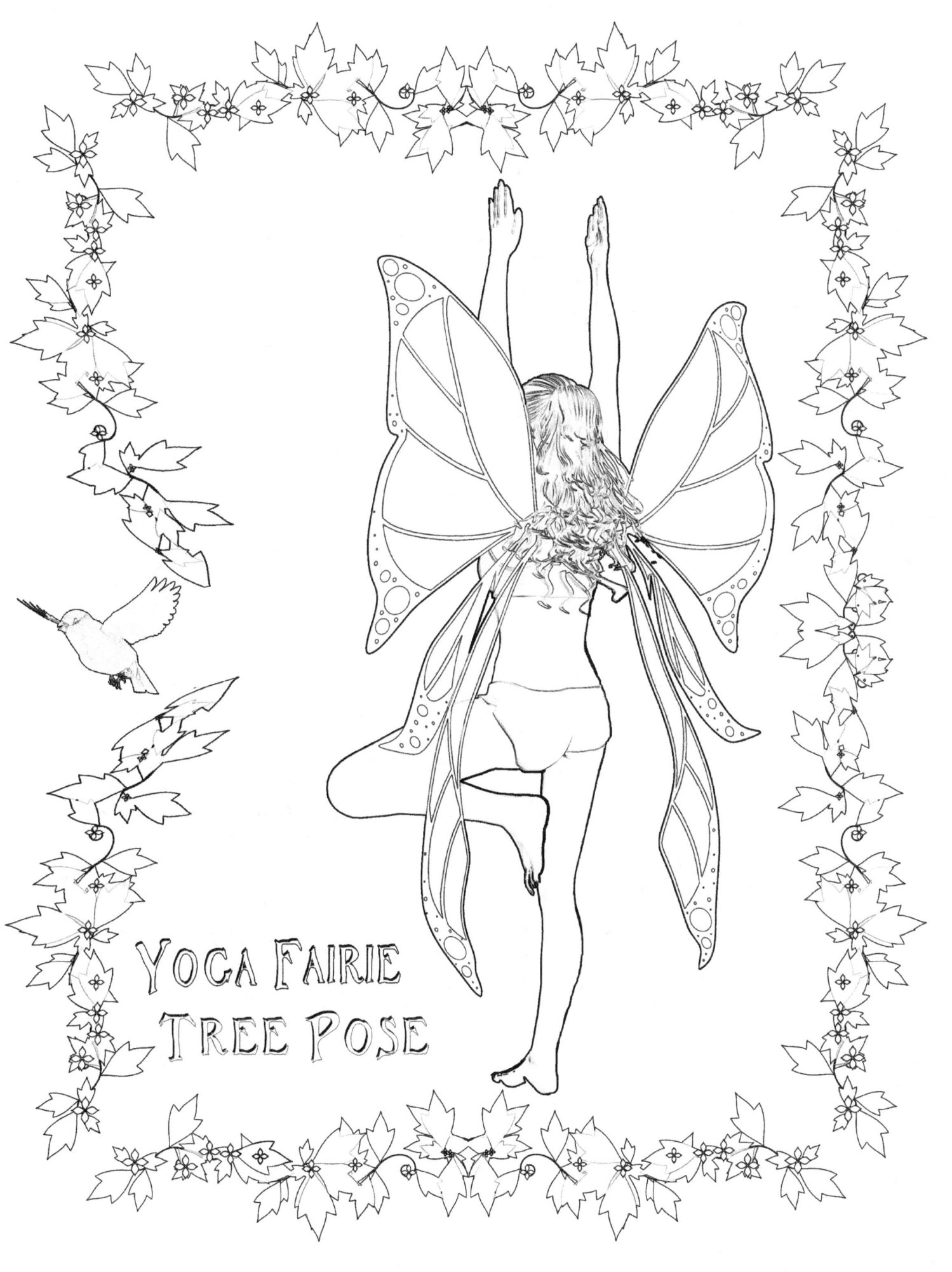

YOGA FAIRIE
TREE POSE

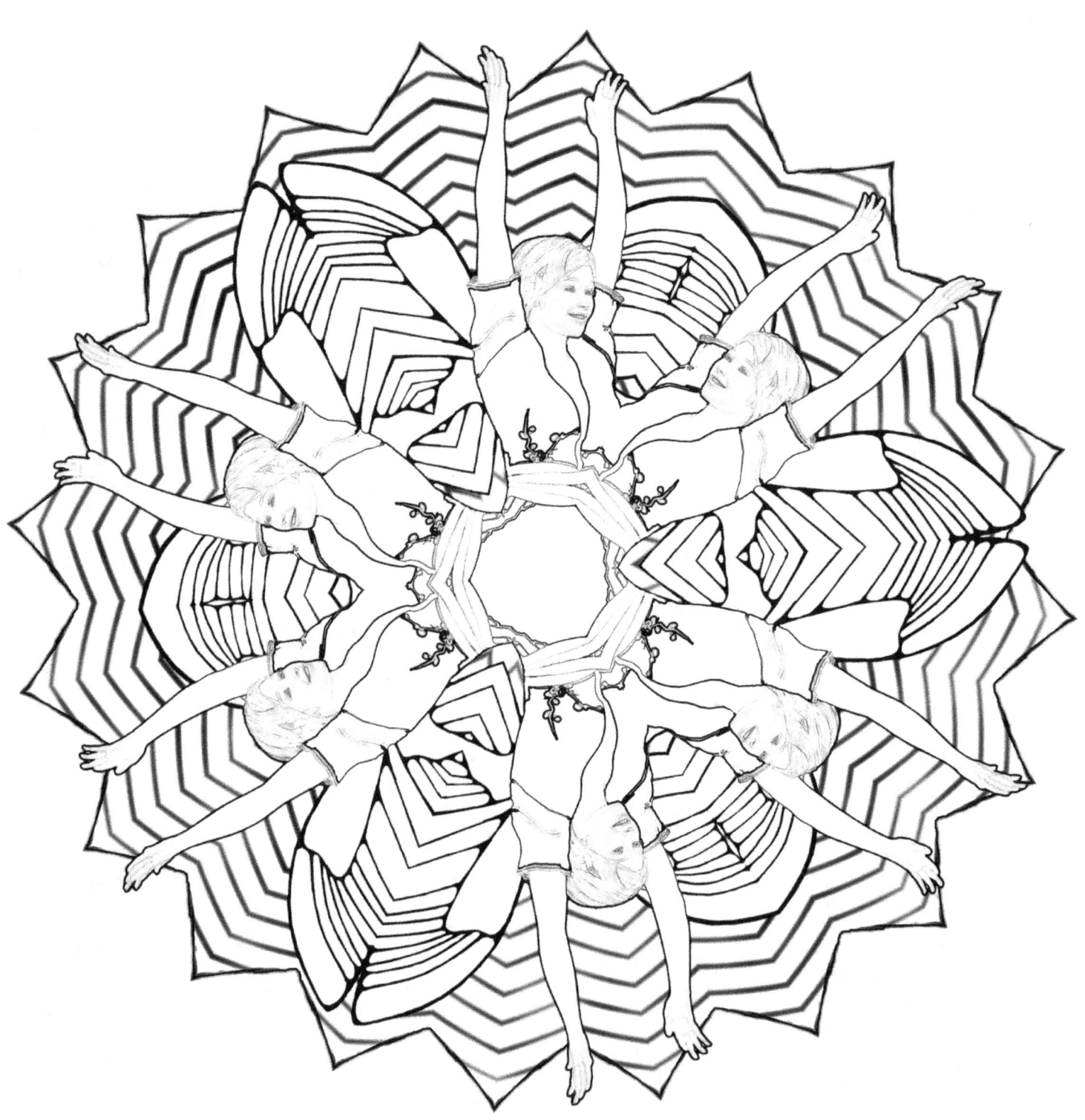

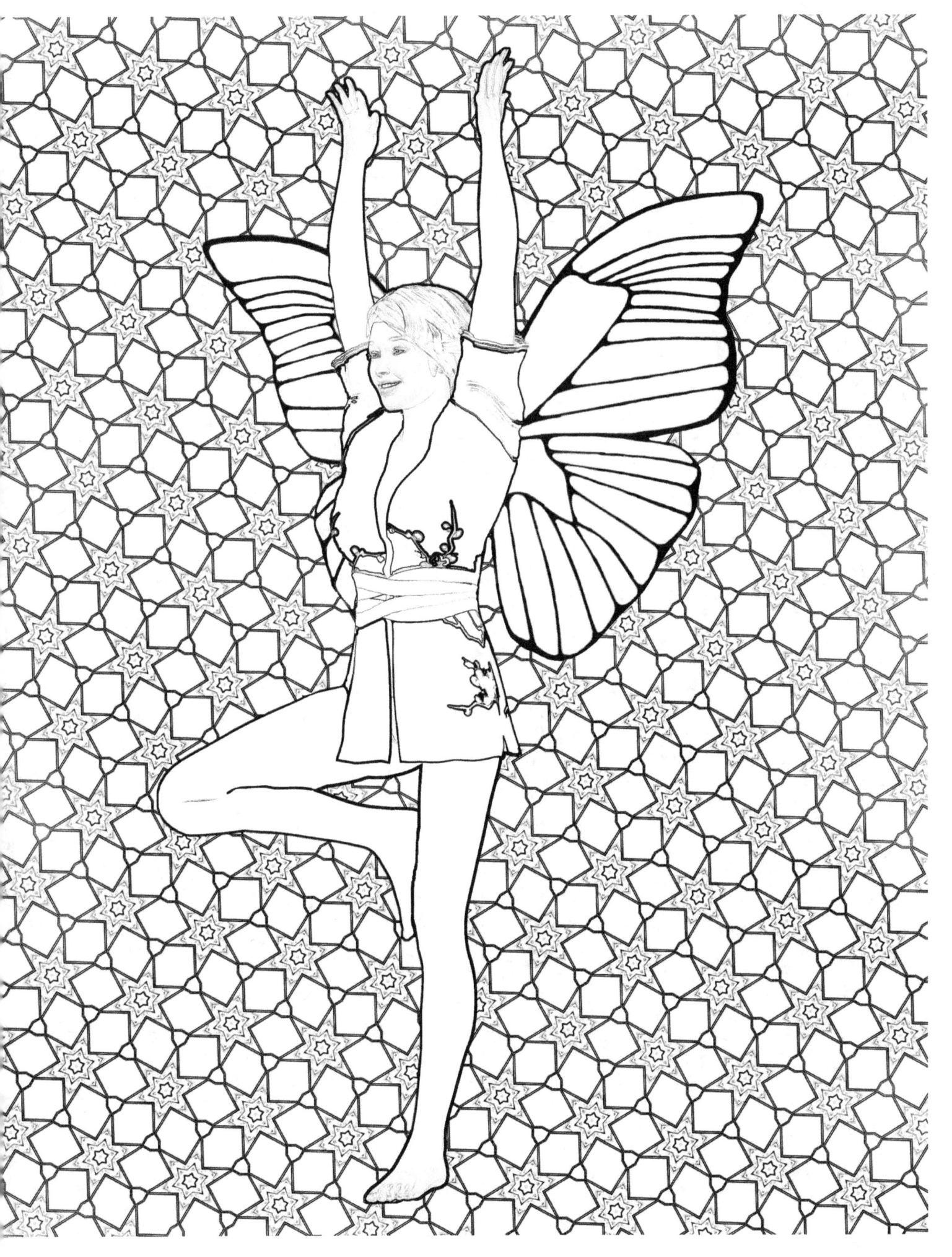

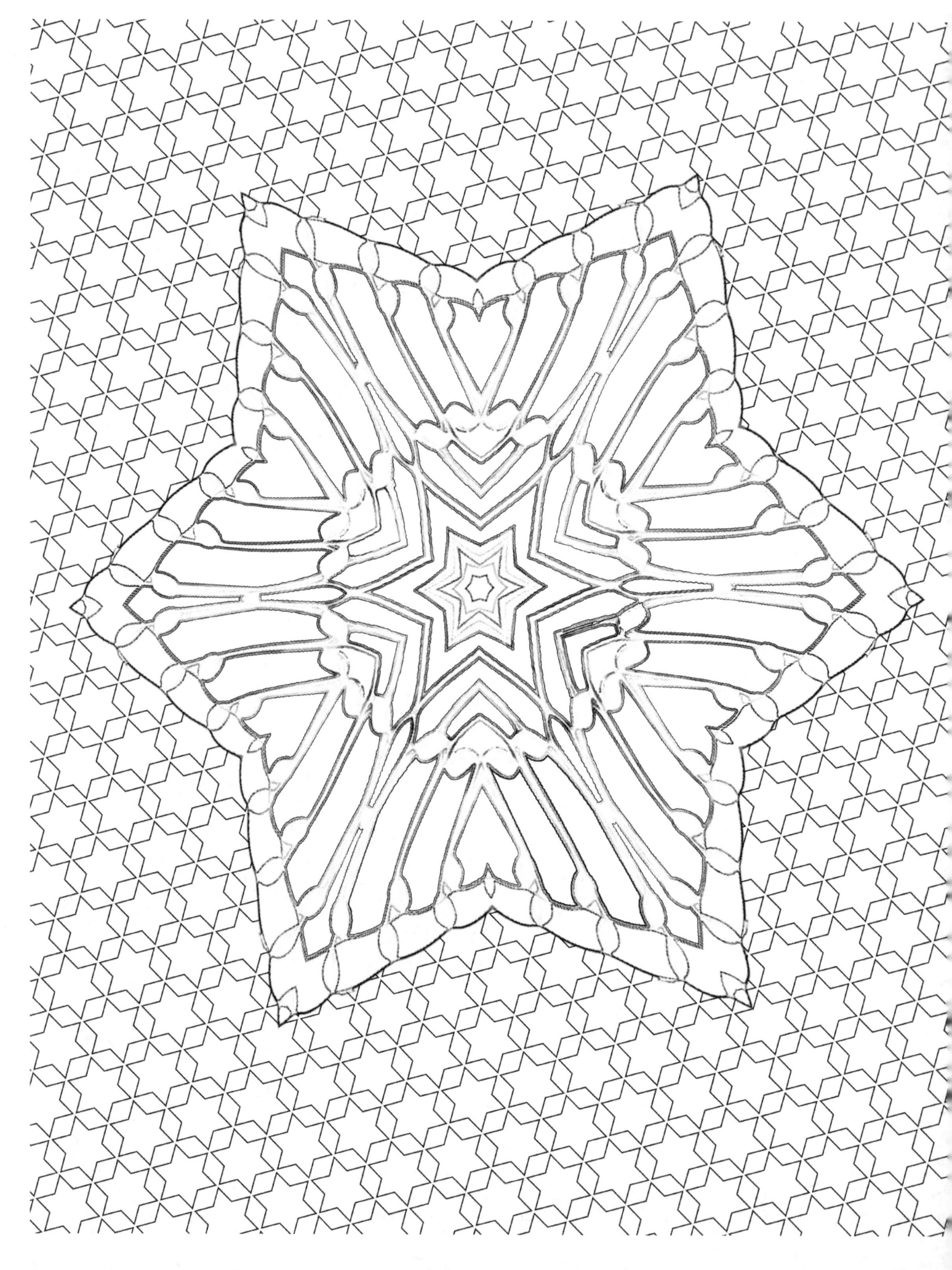

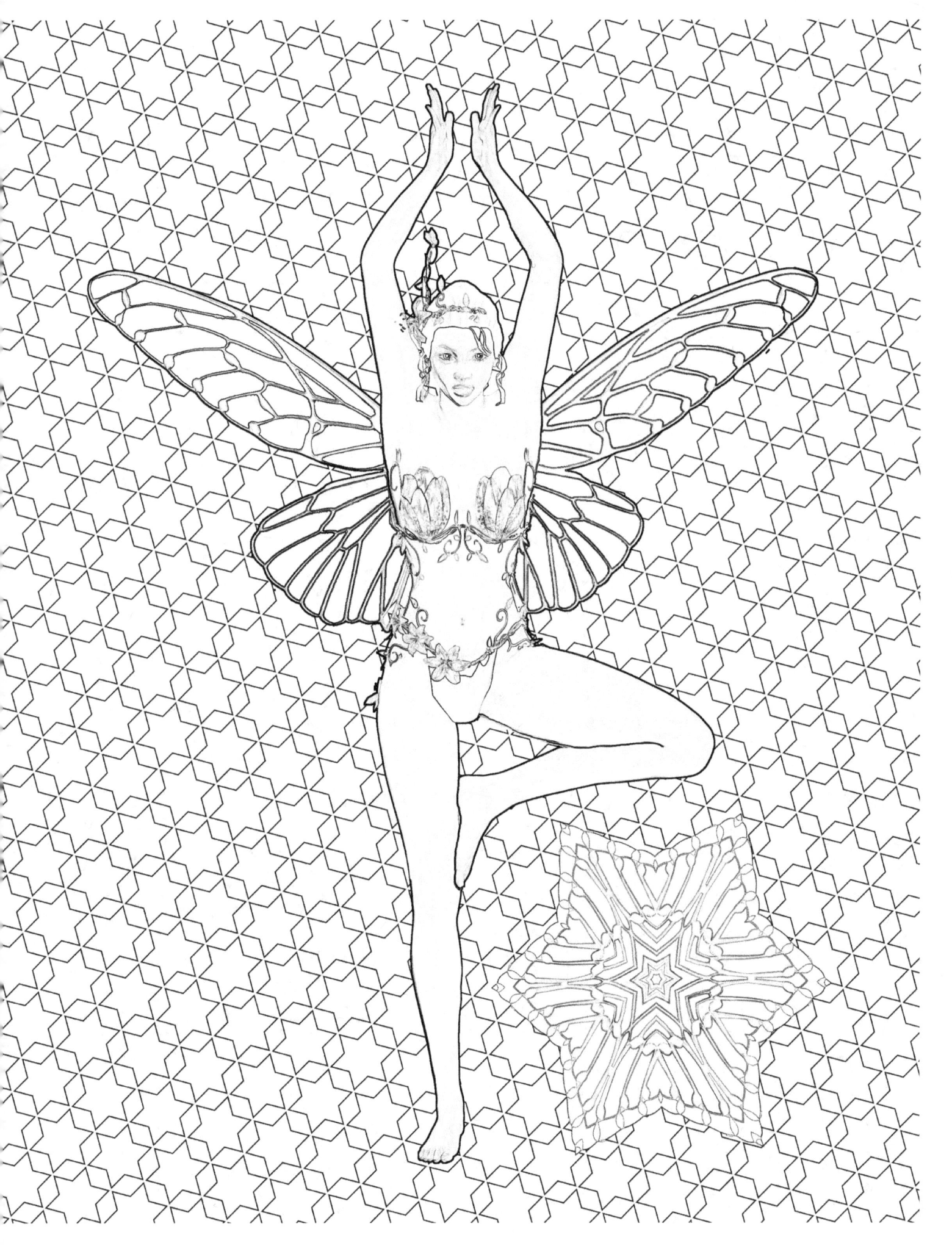

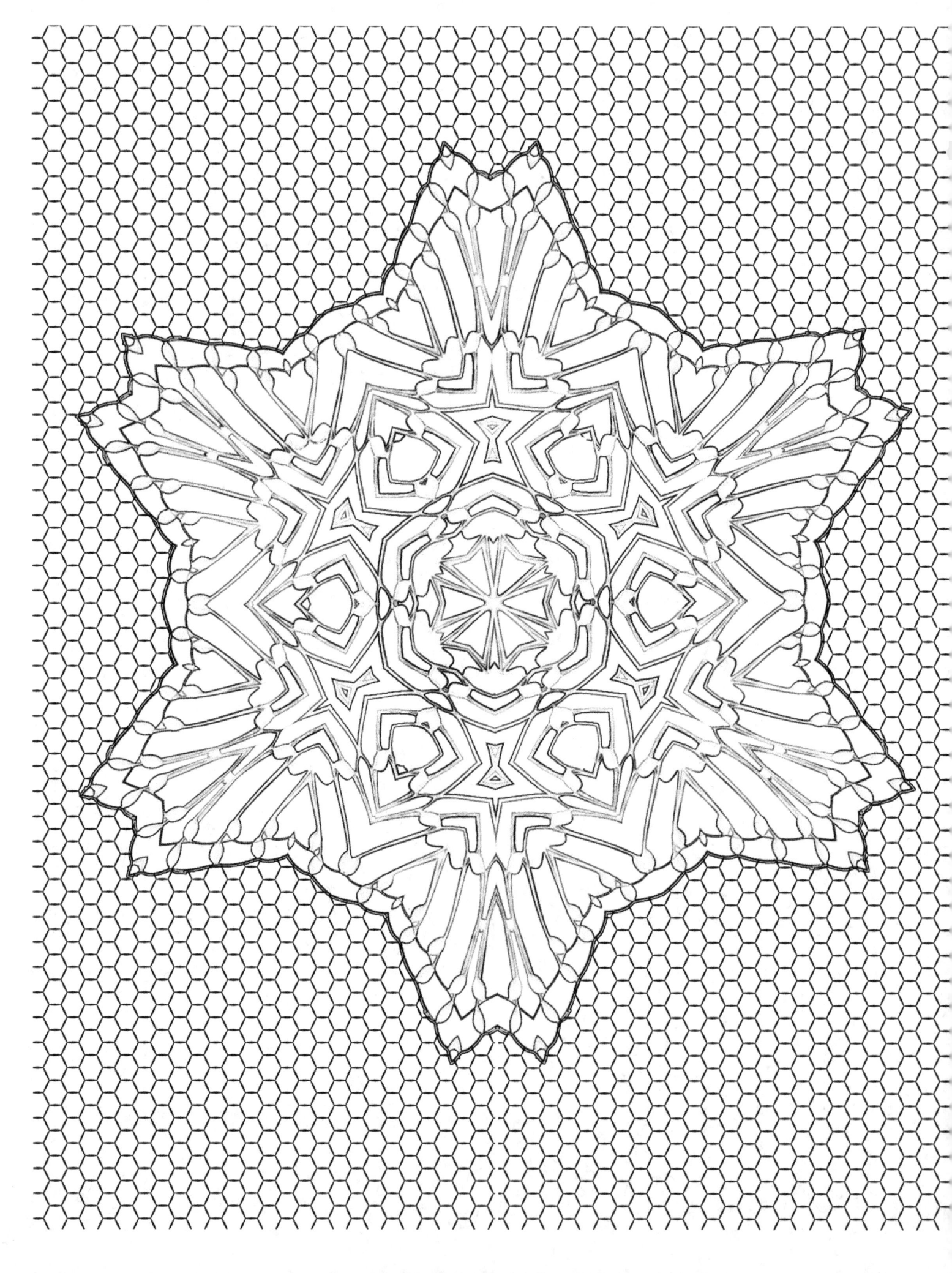

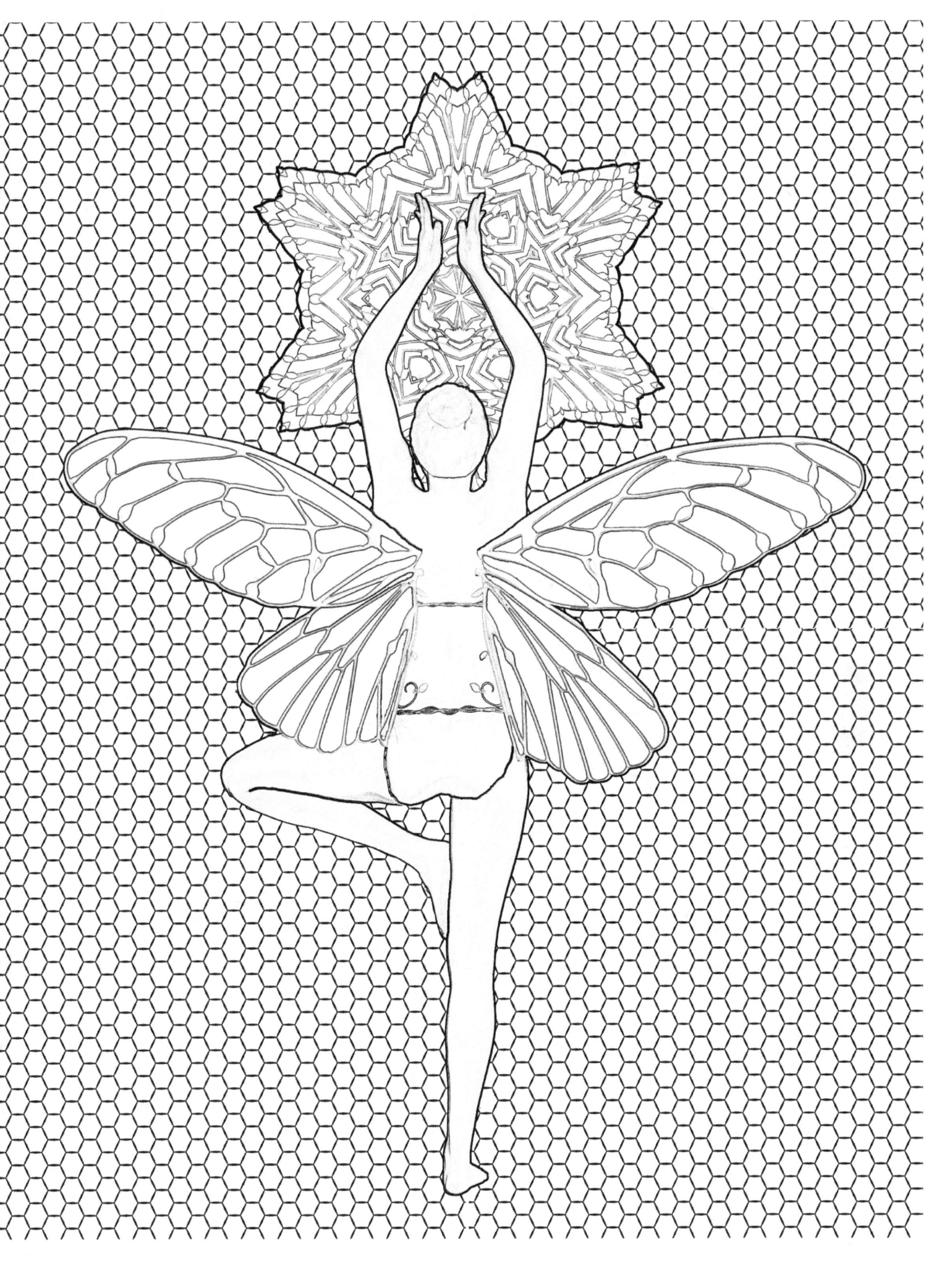

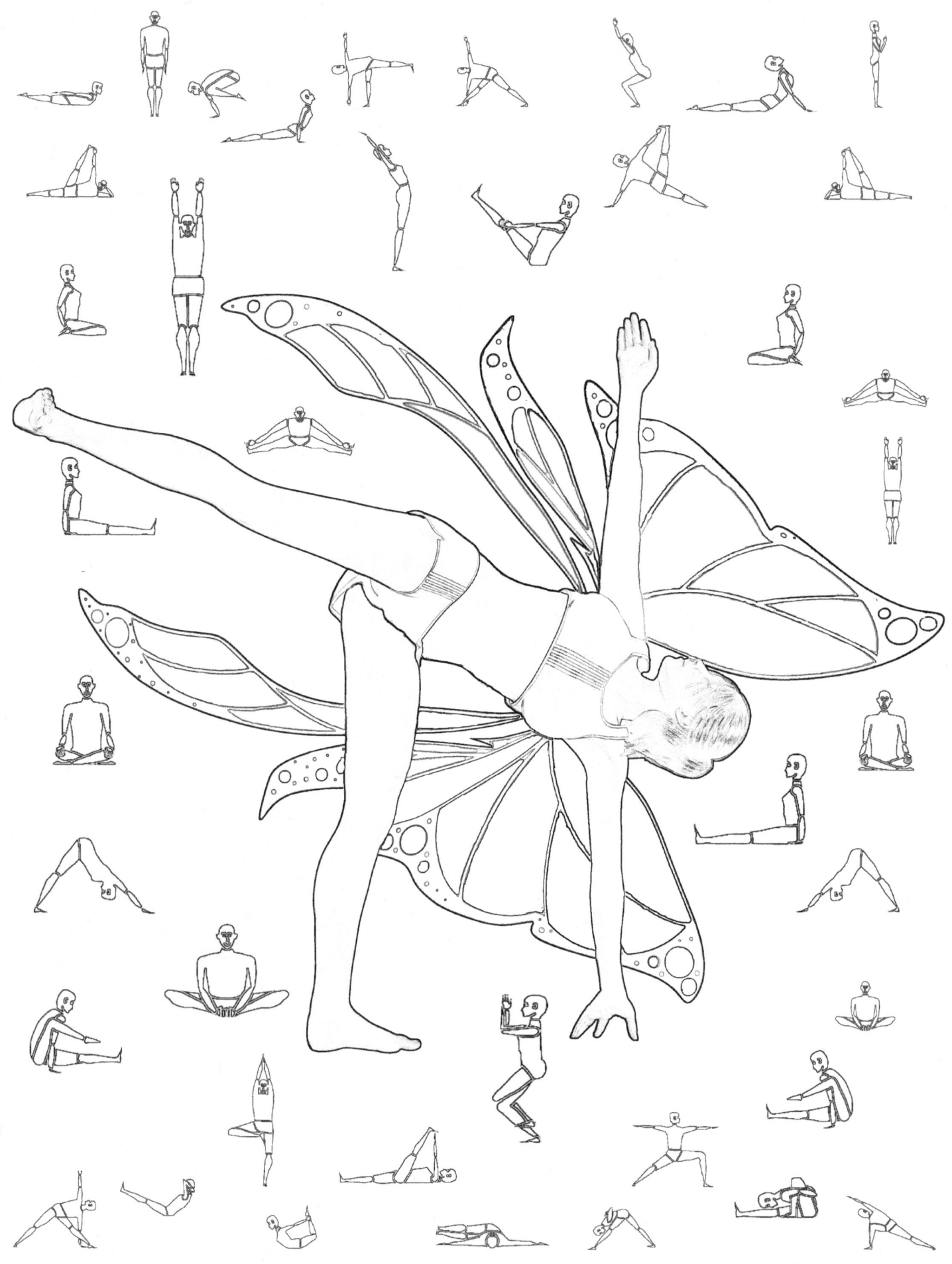

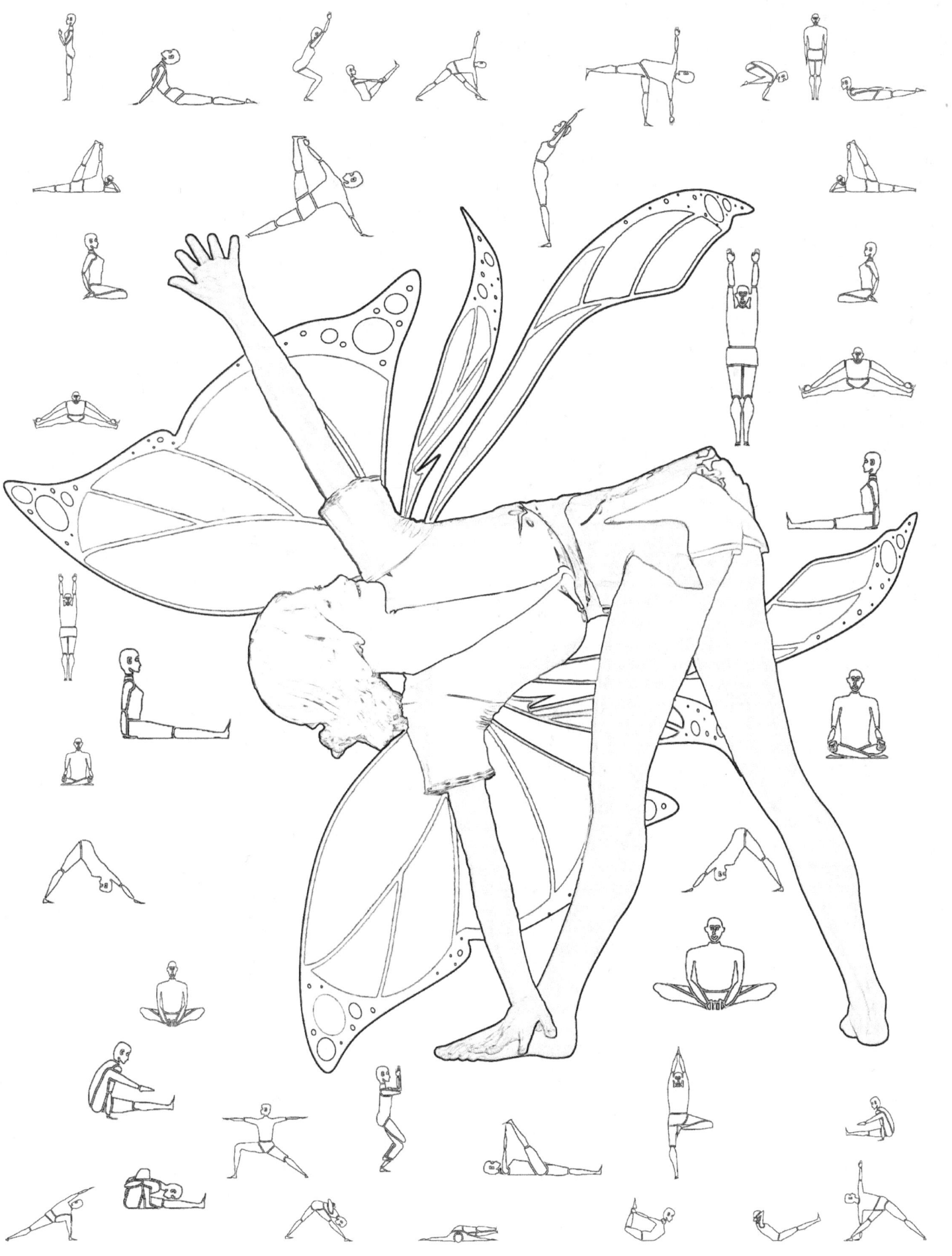

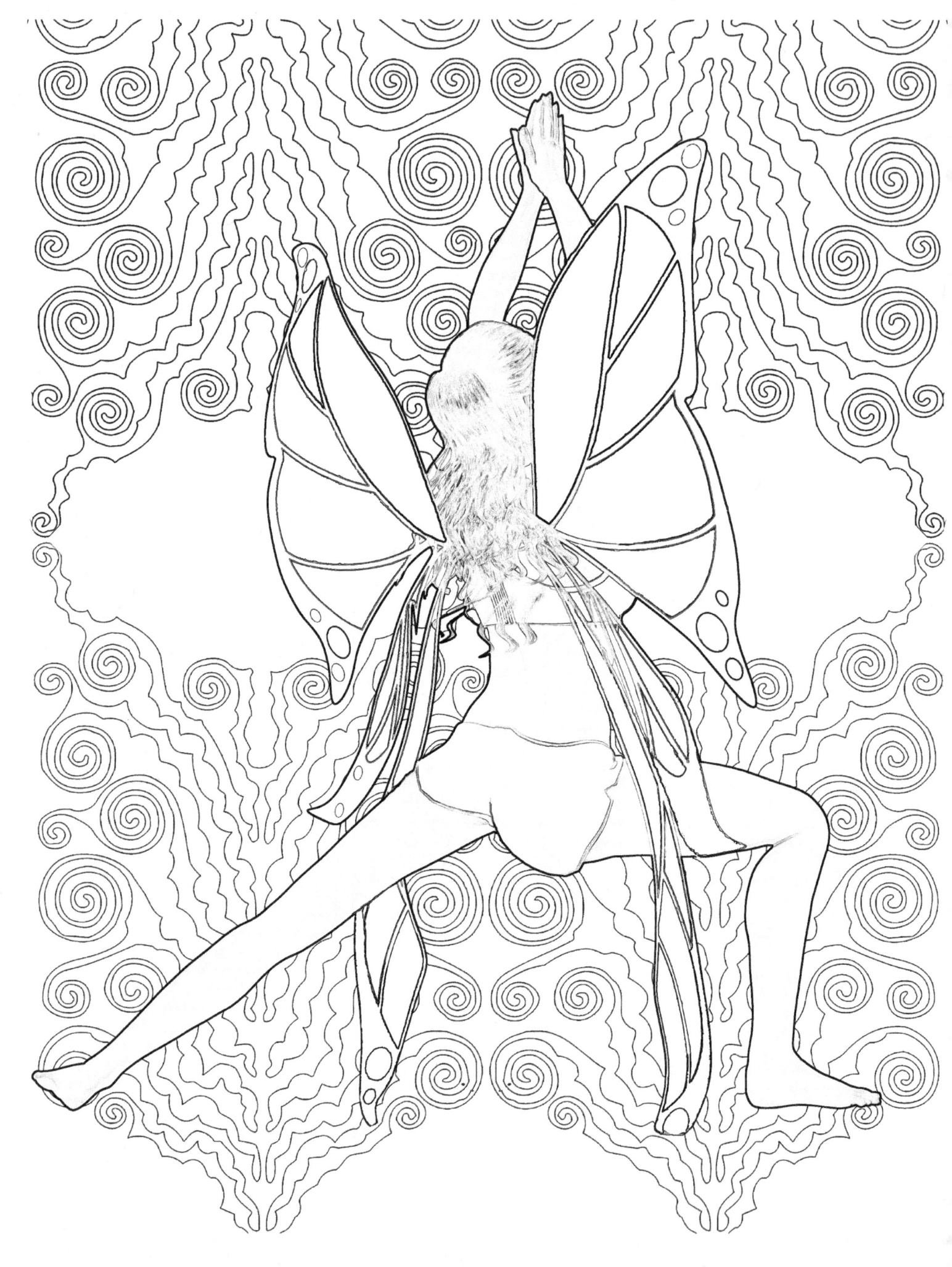

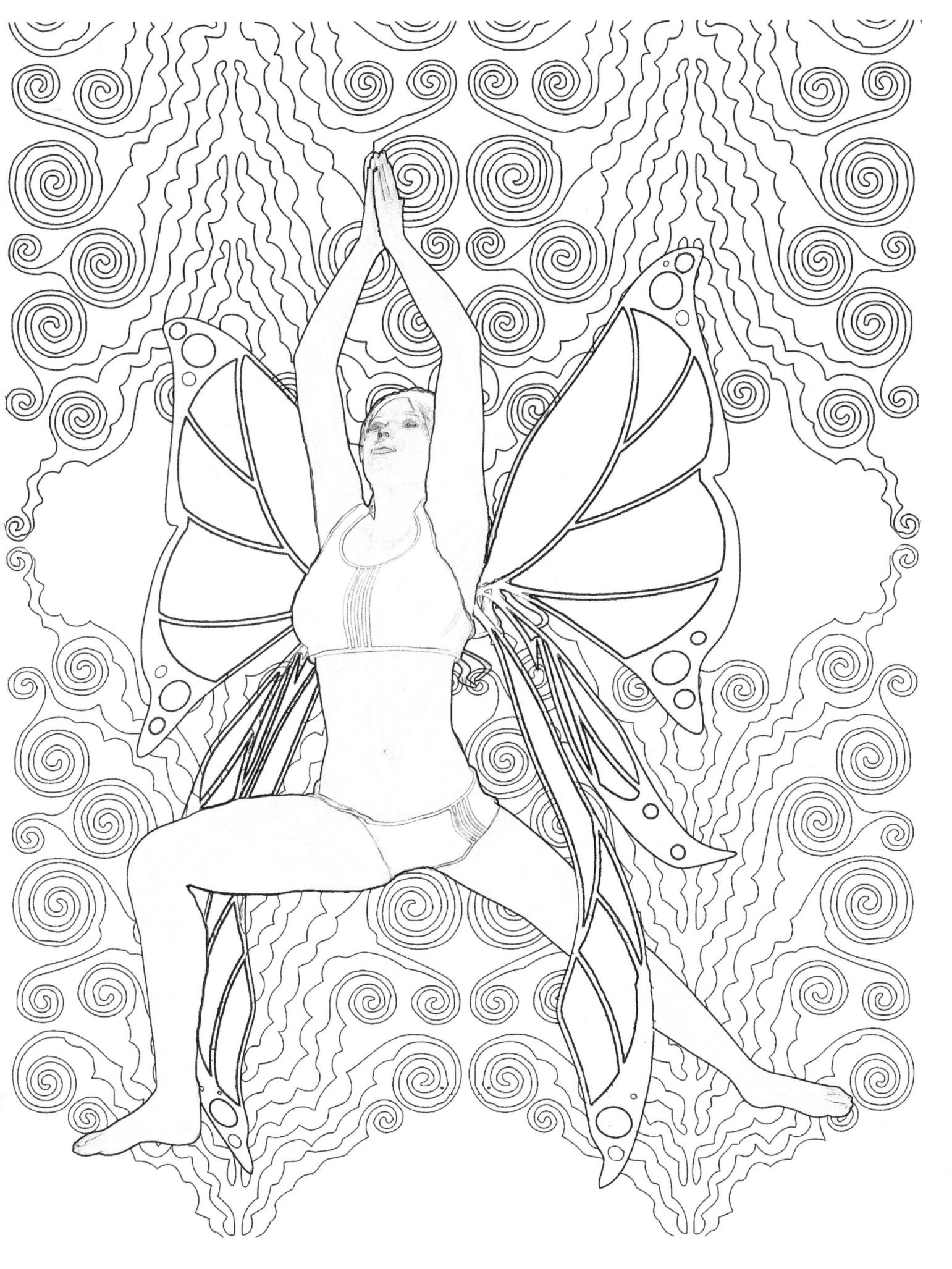

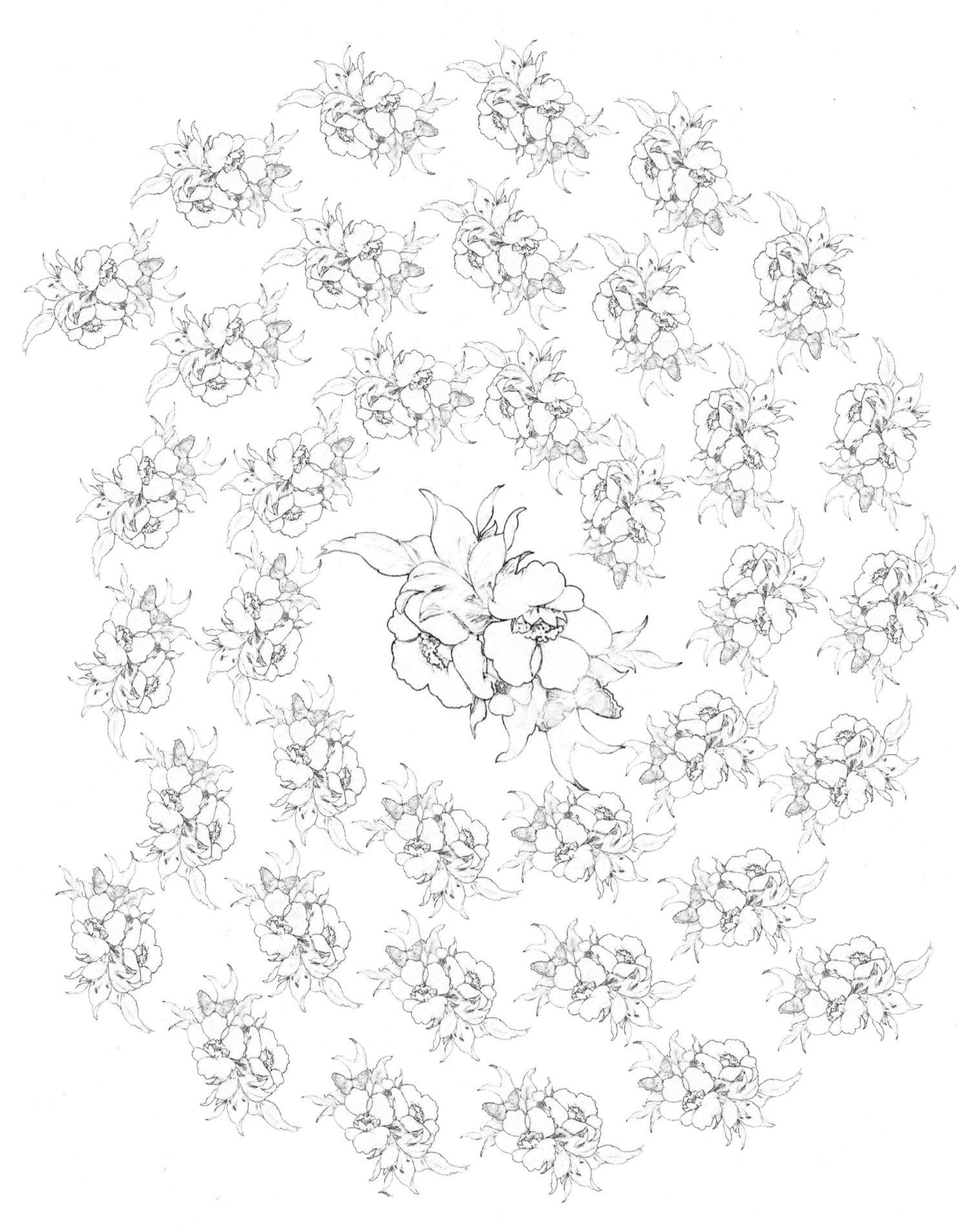

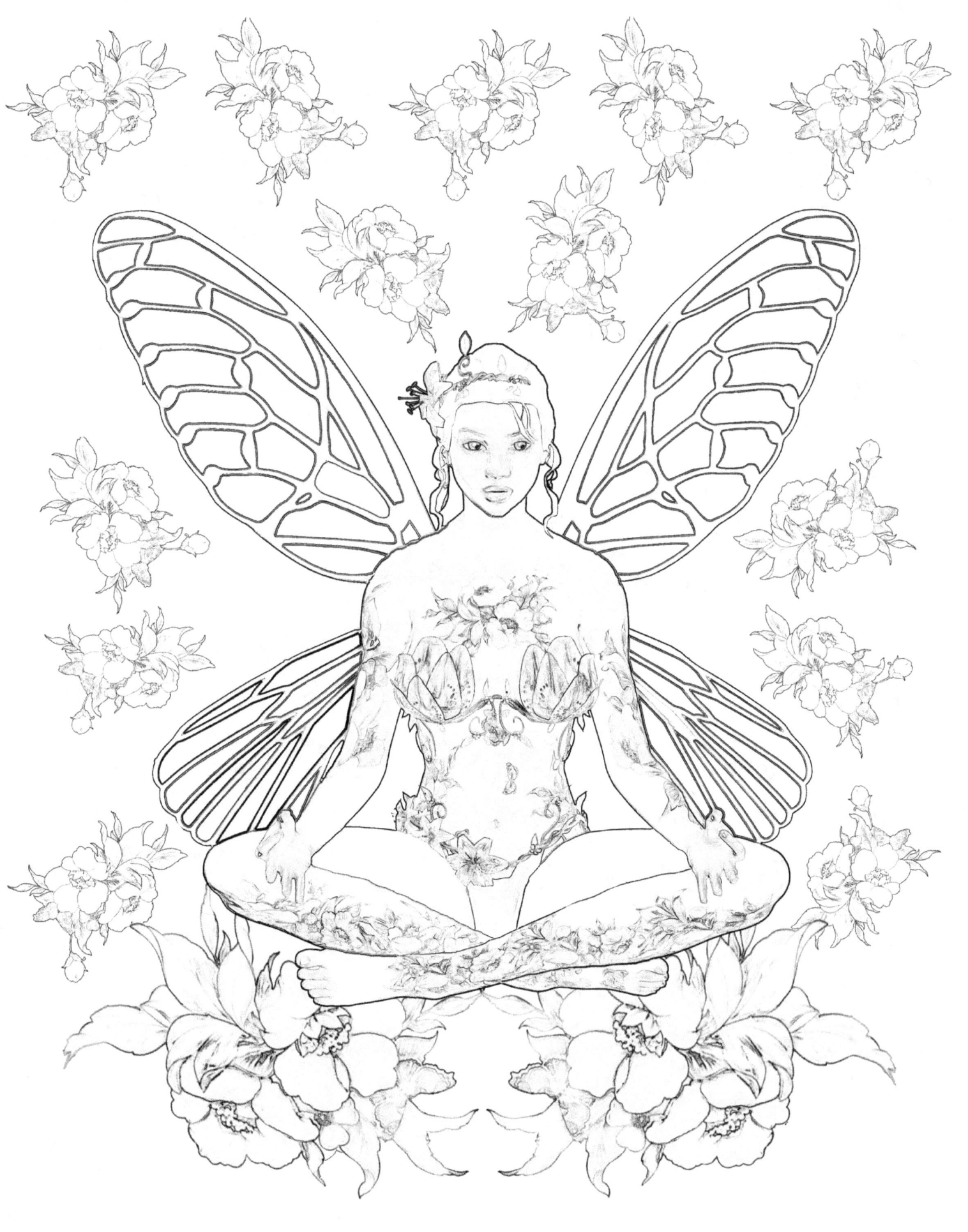

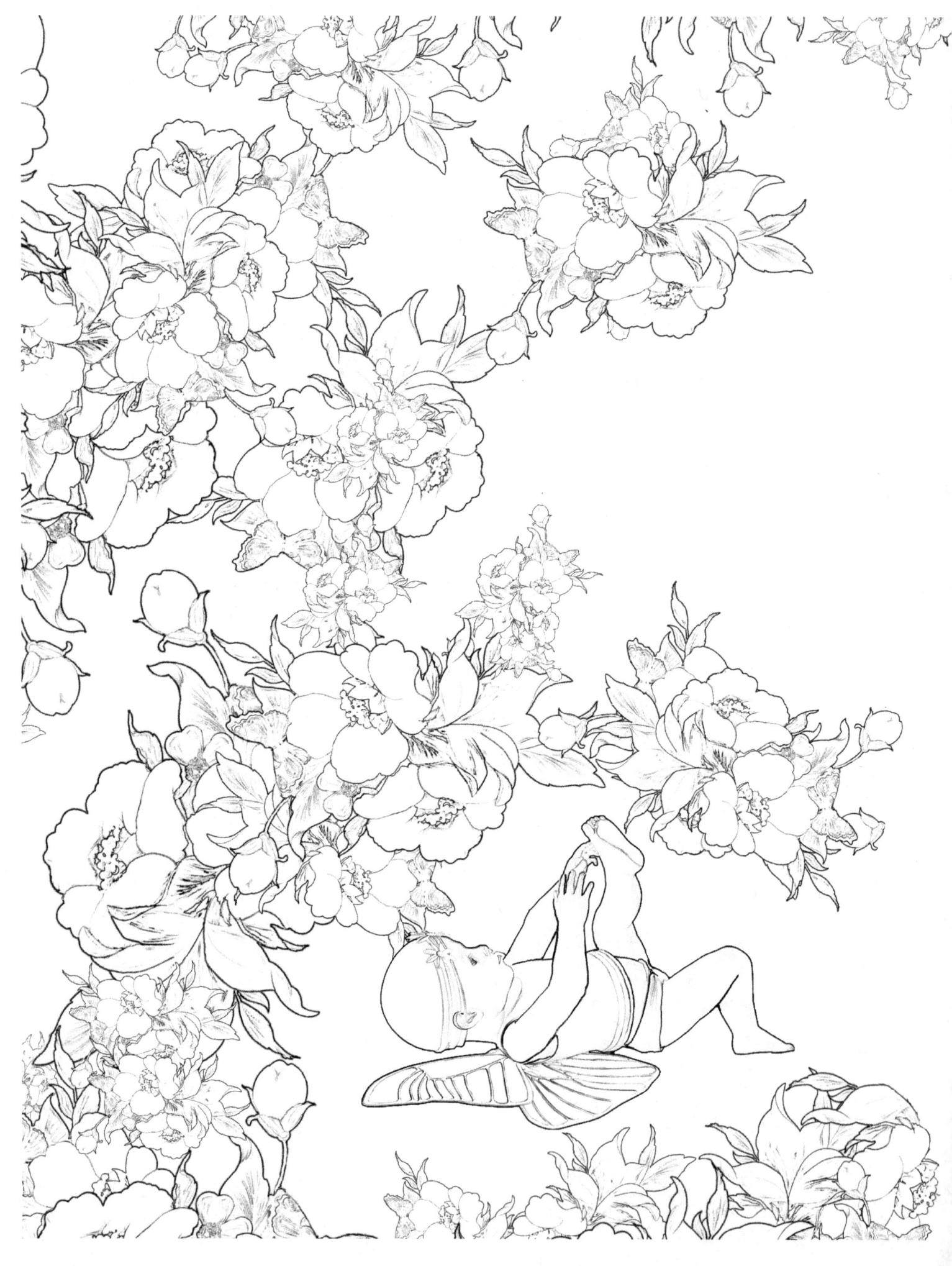

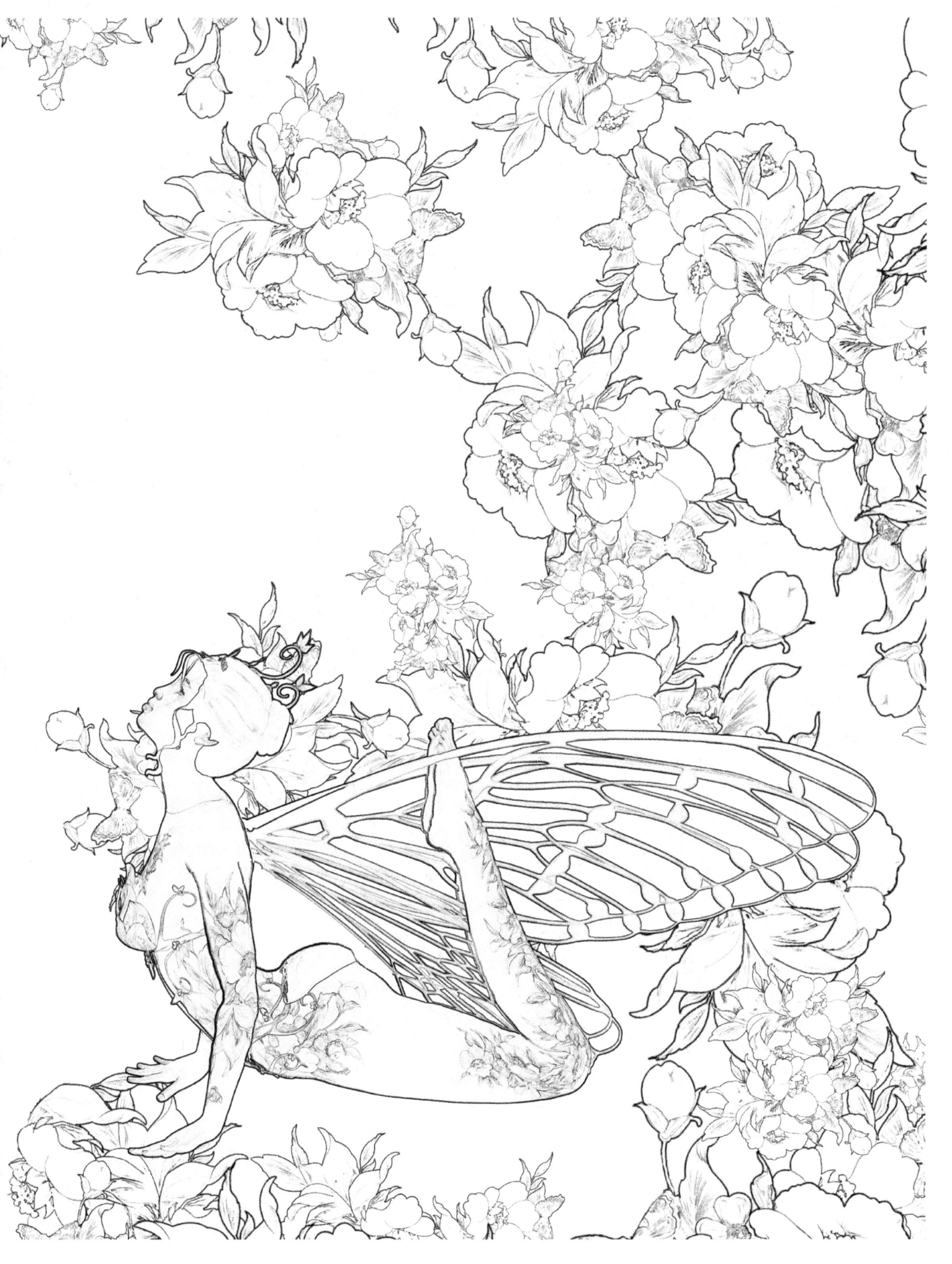

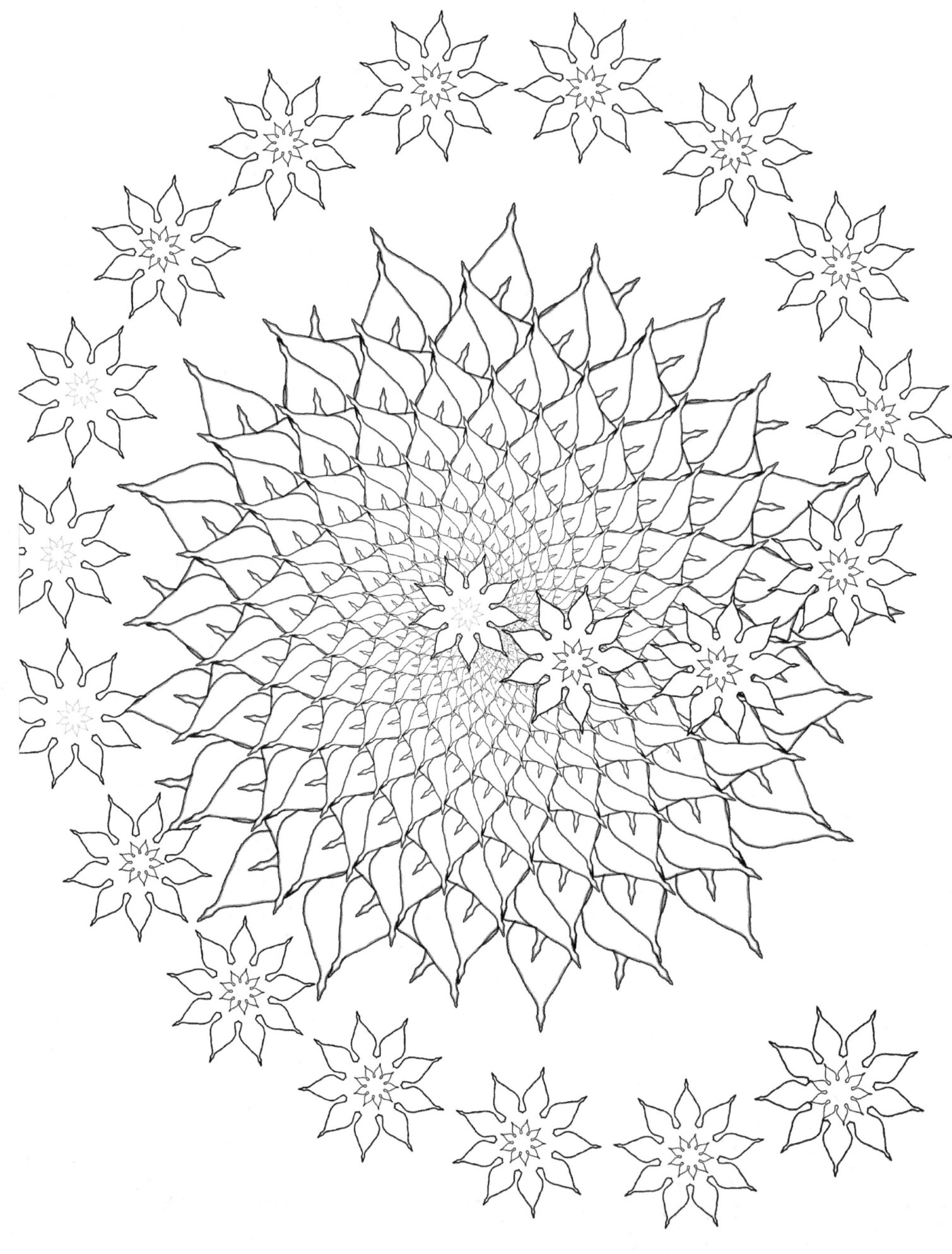

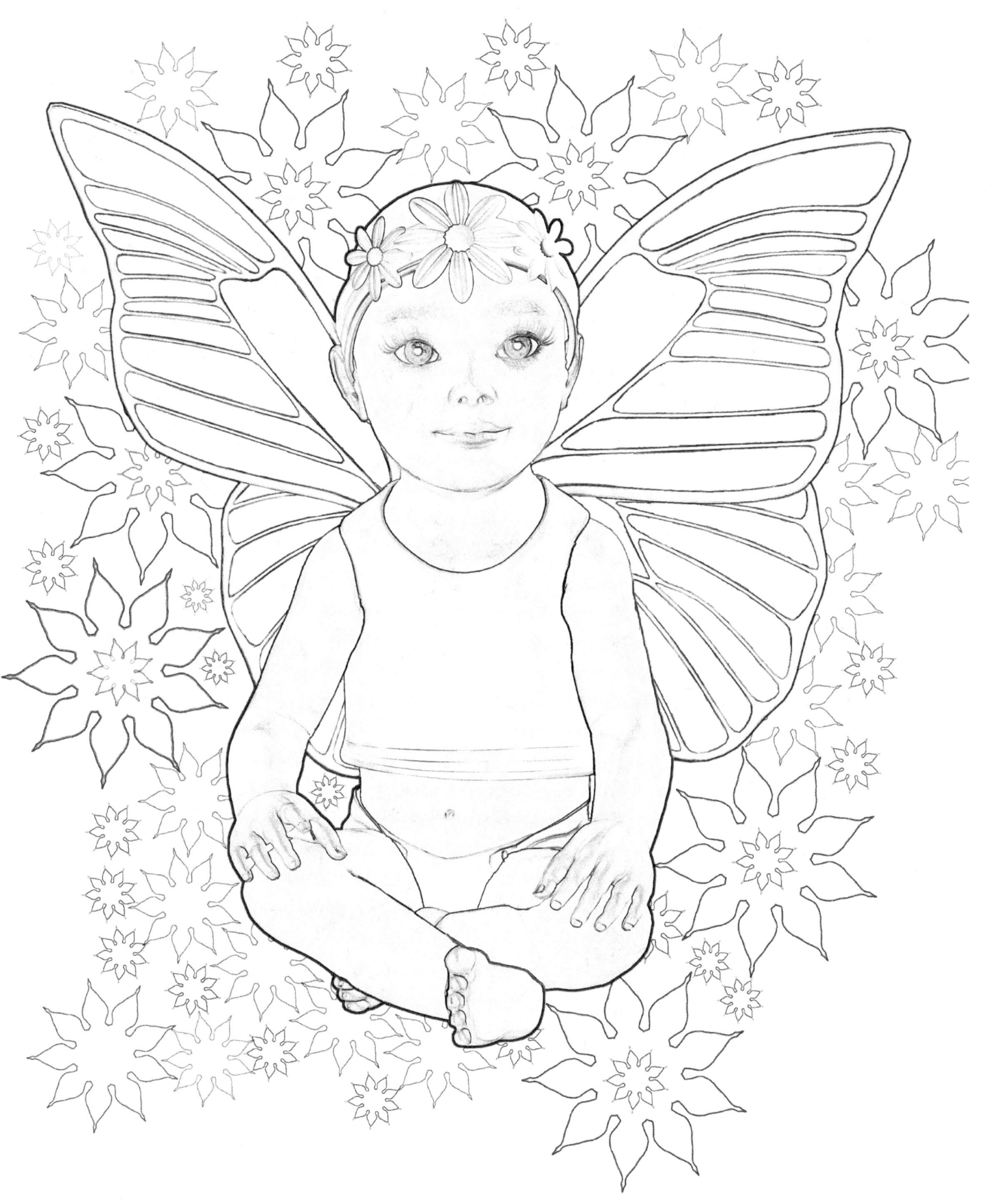

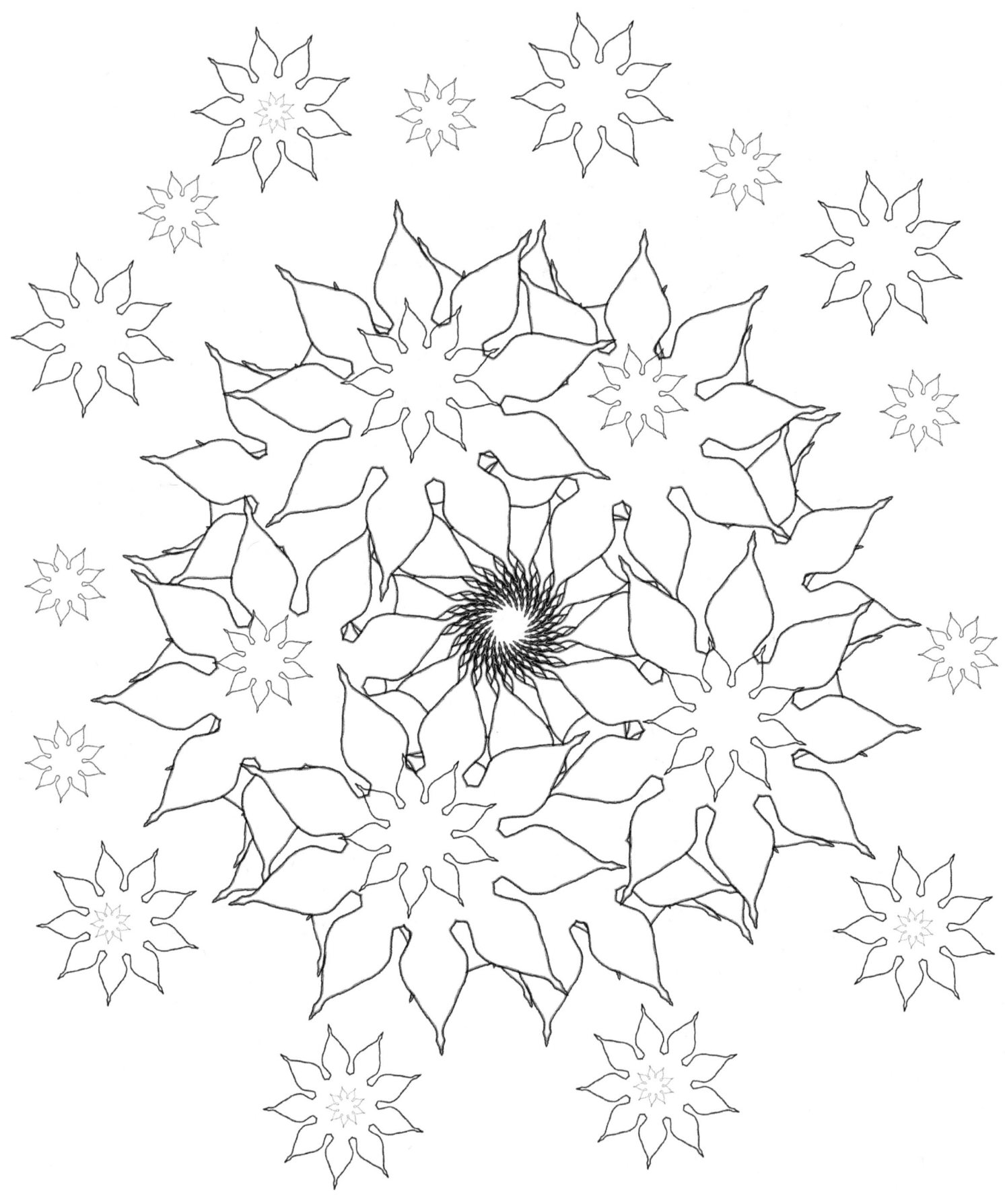

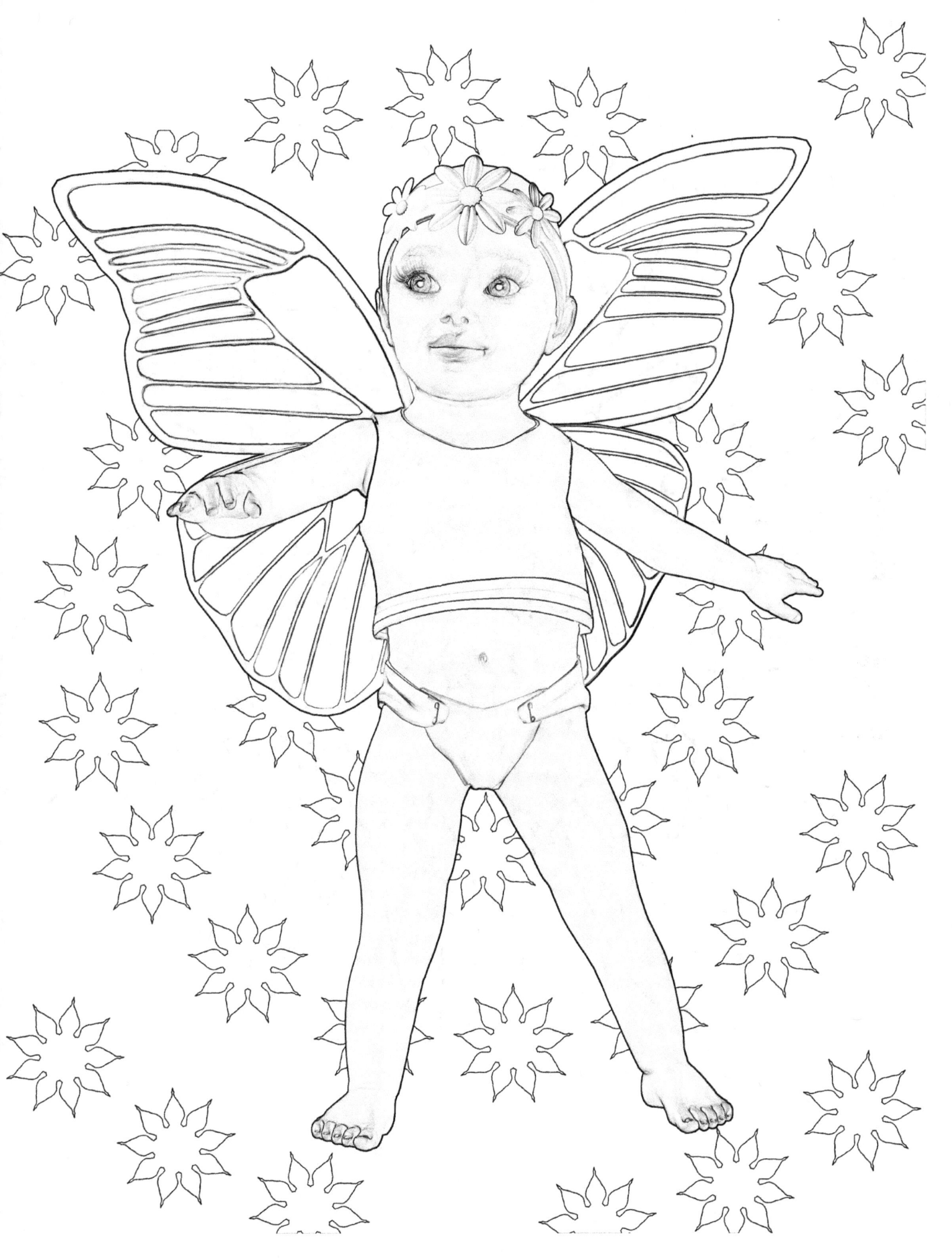

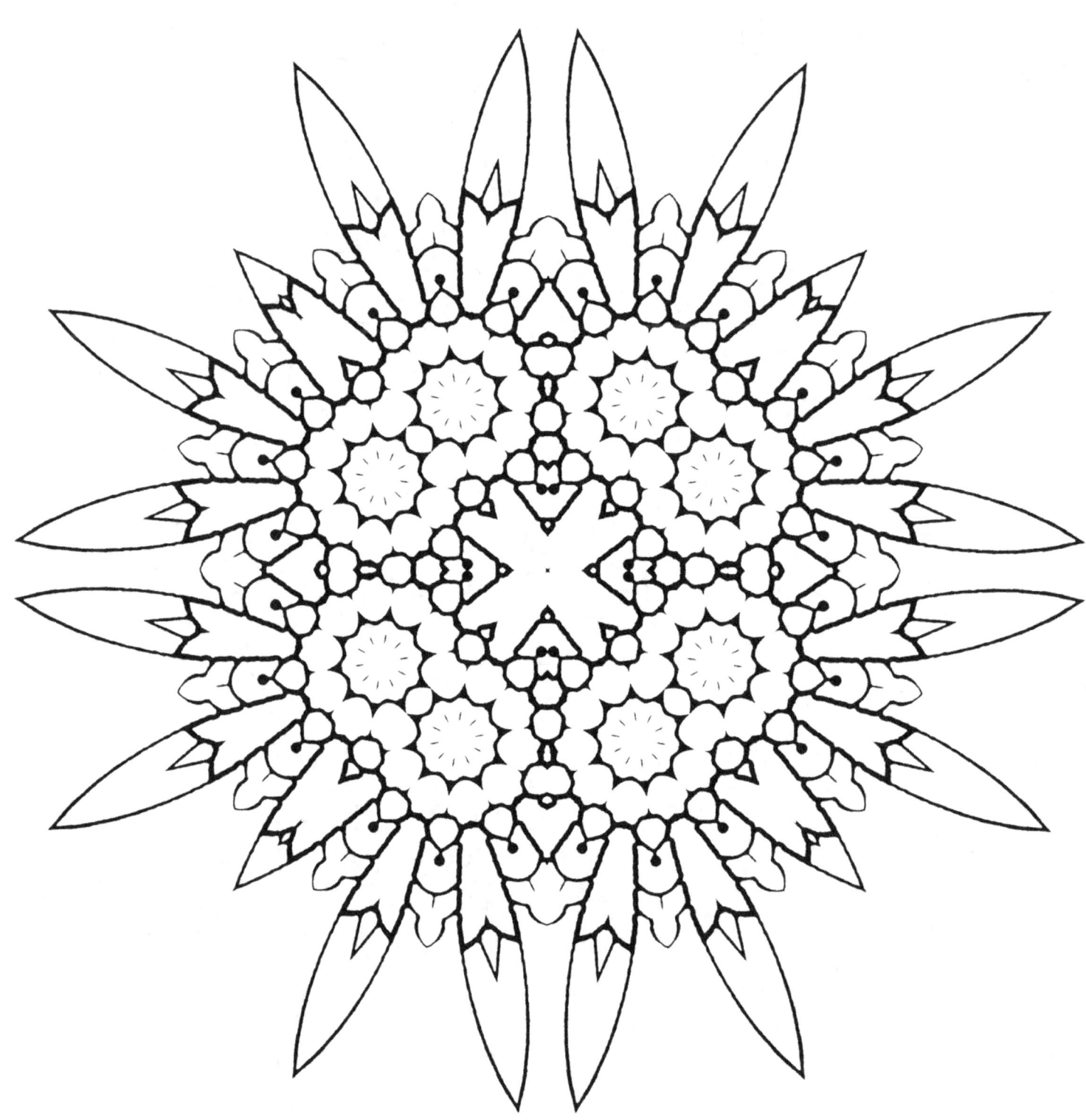

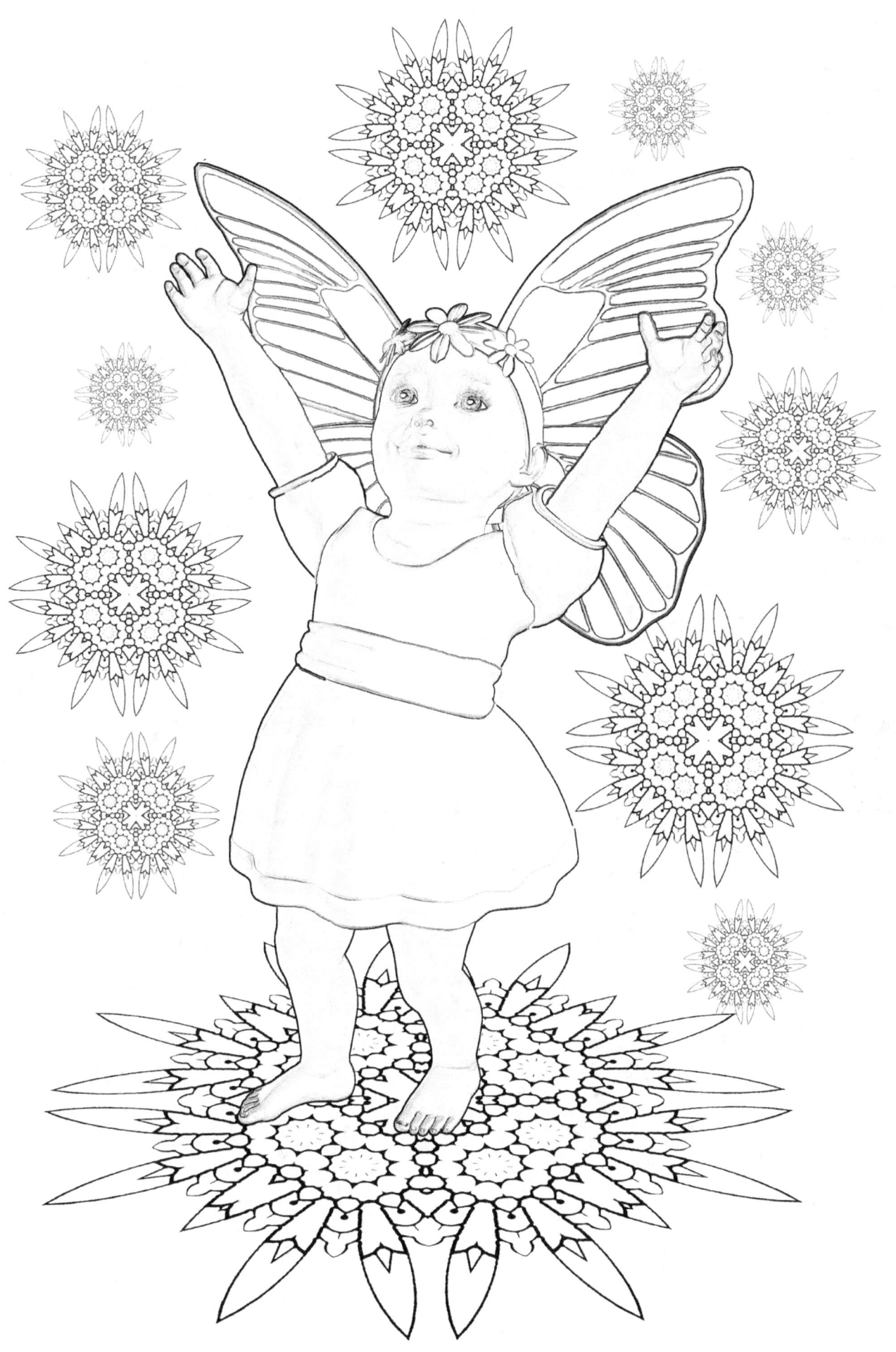

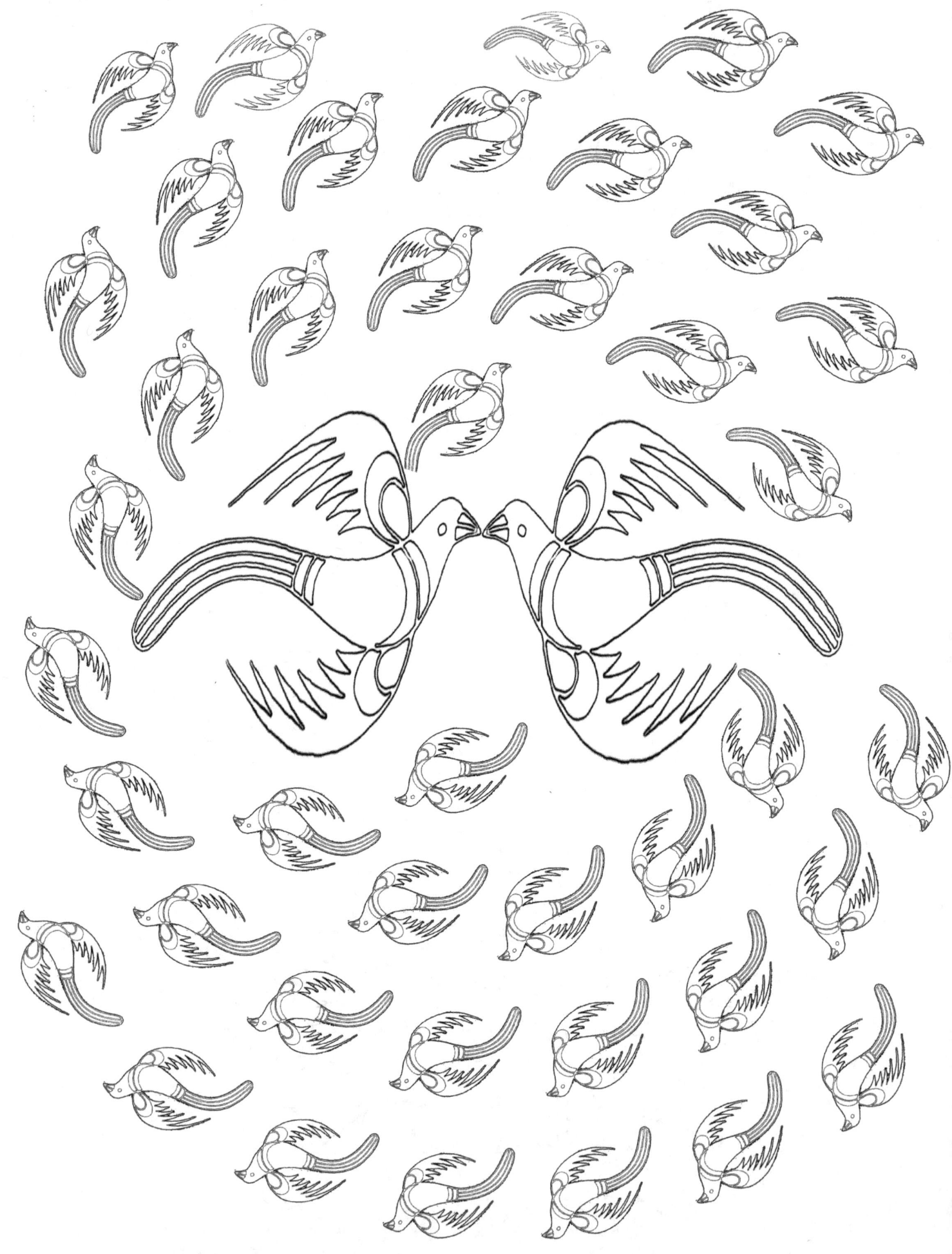

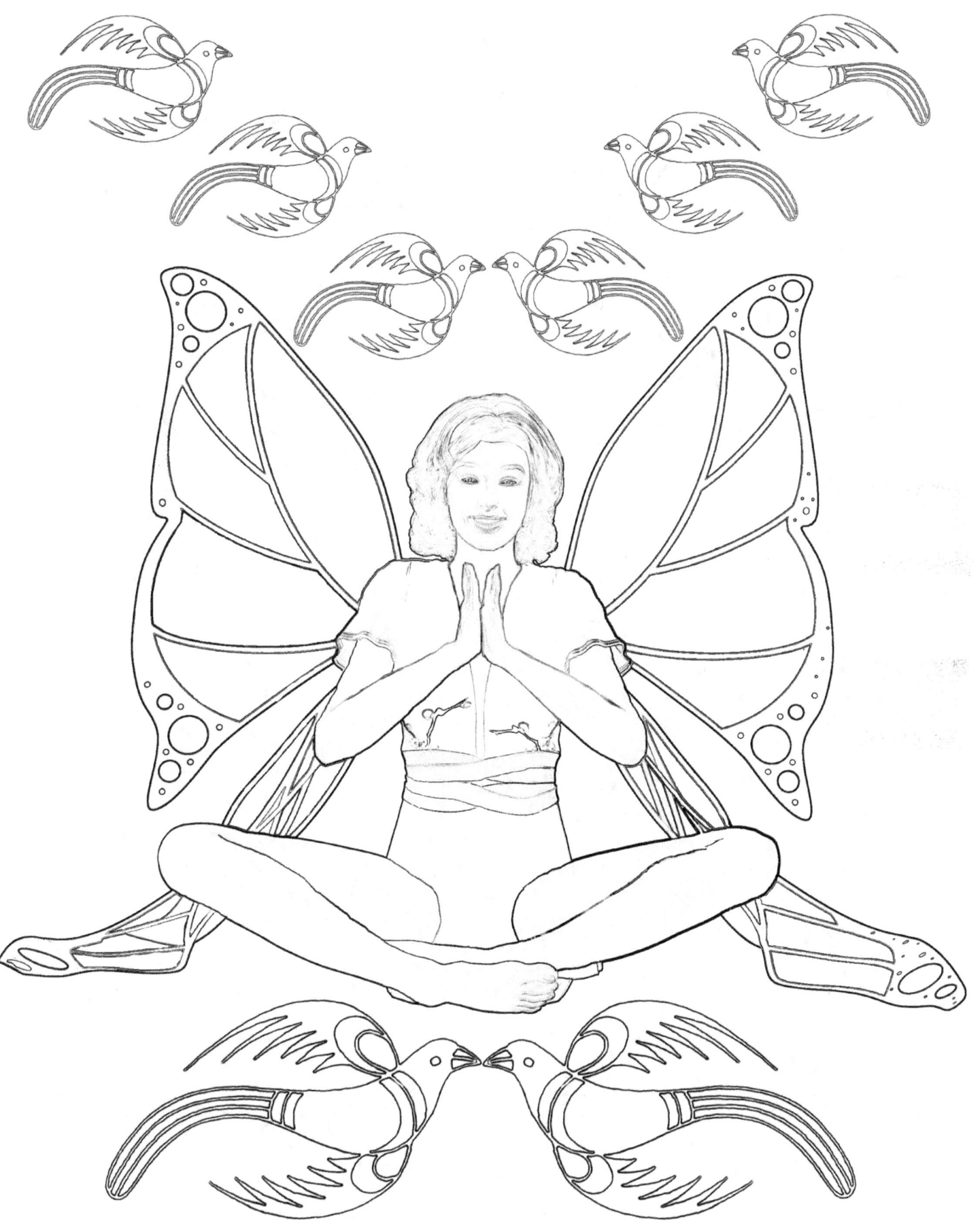

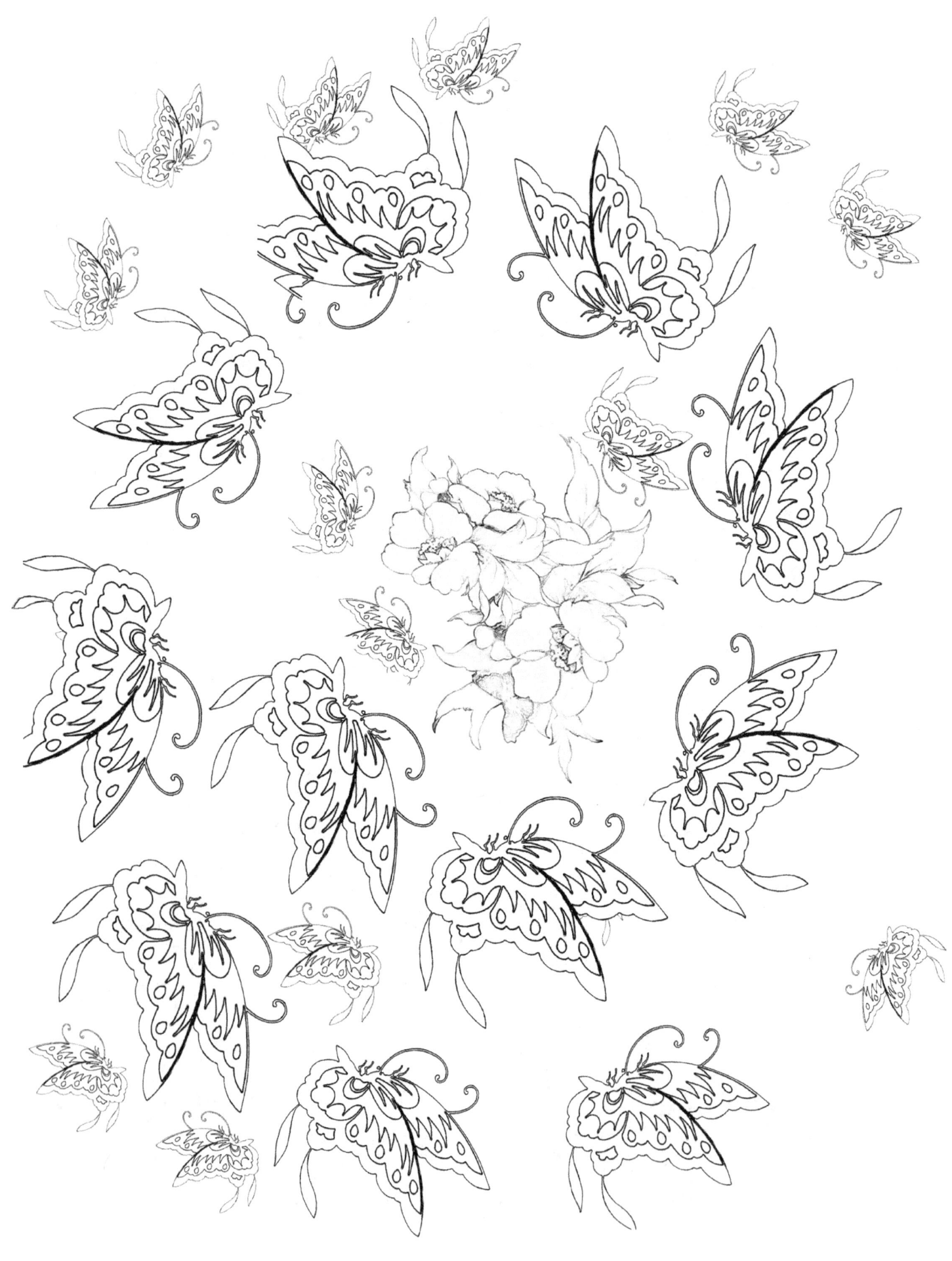

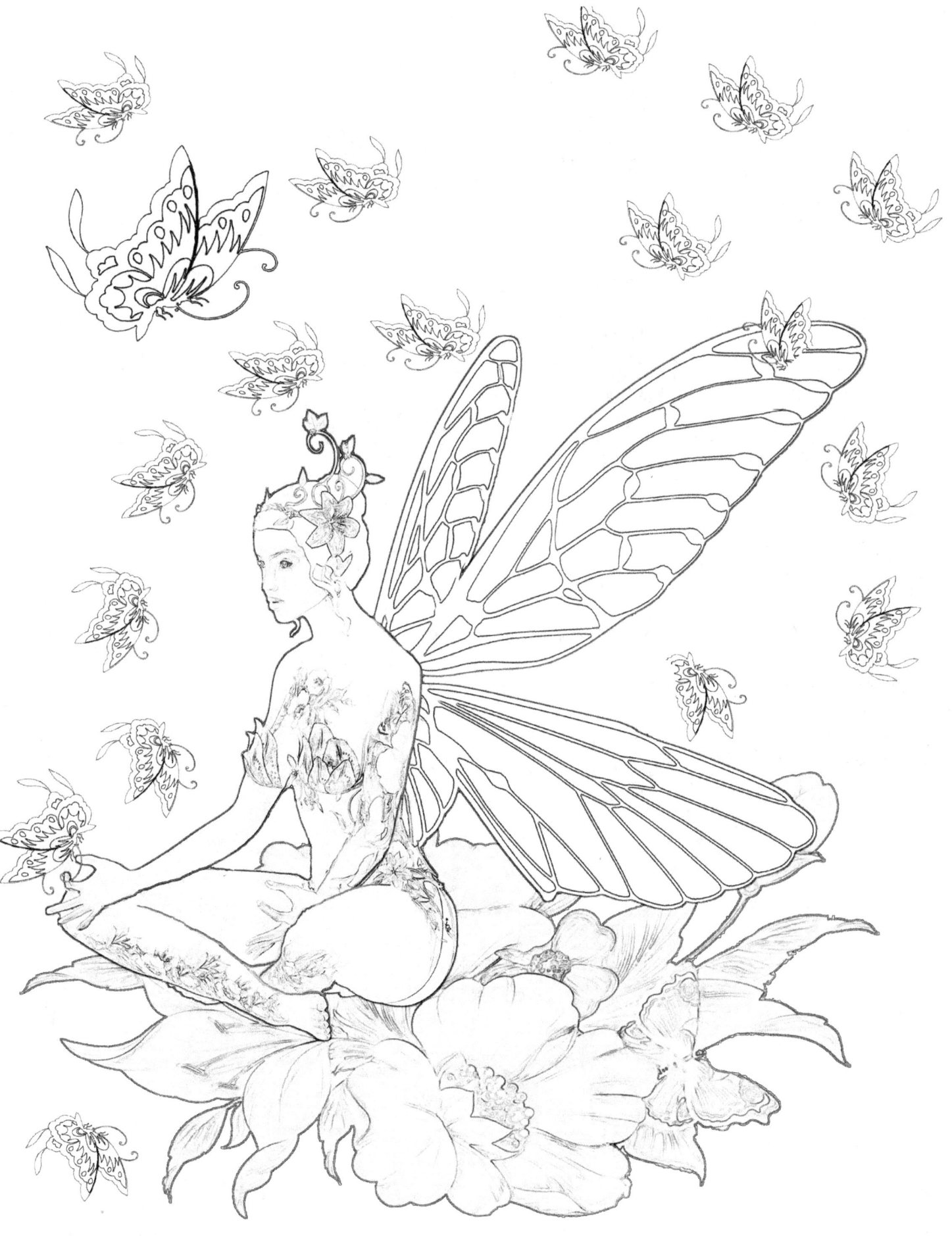

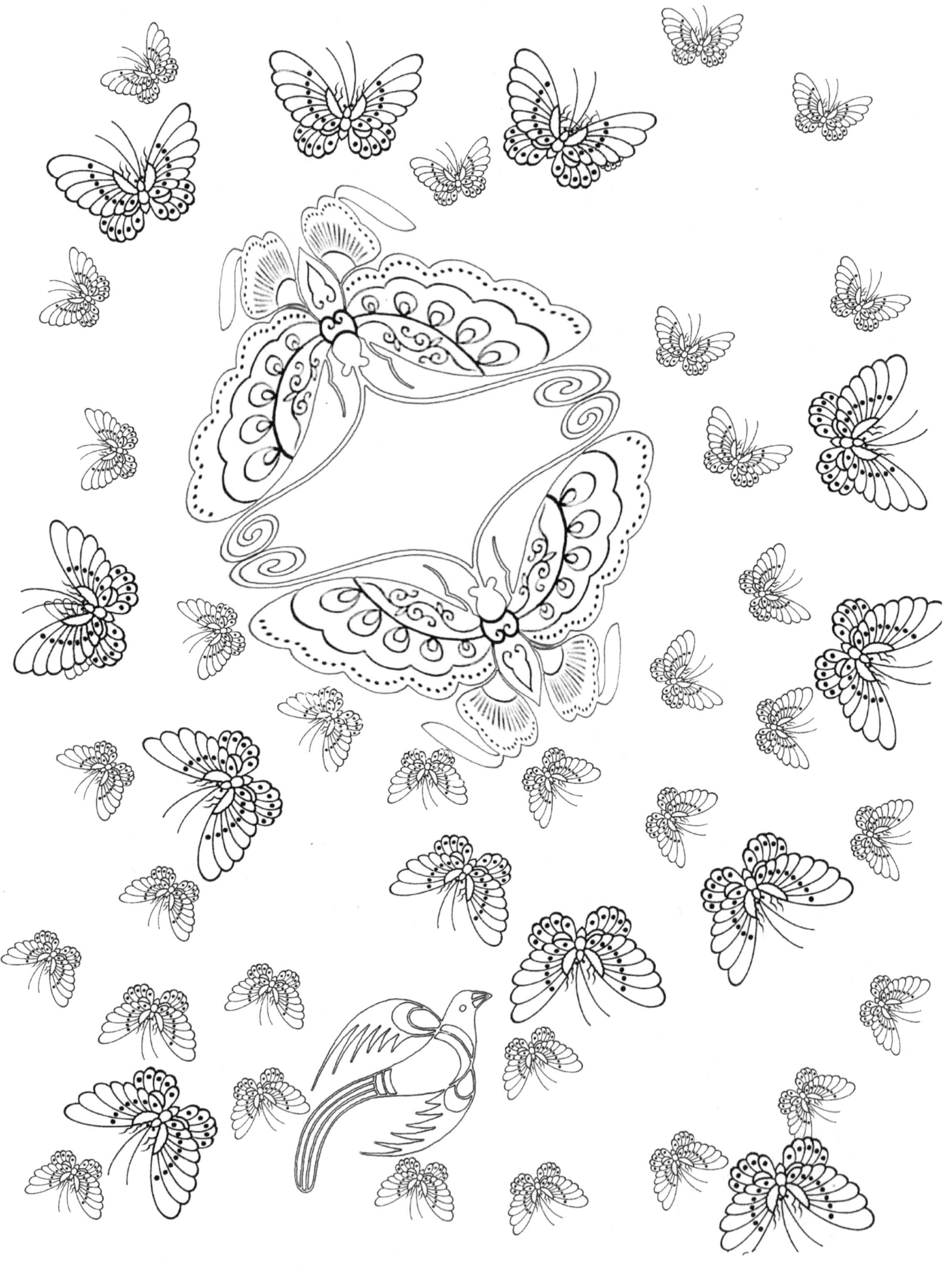

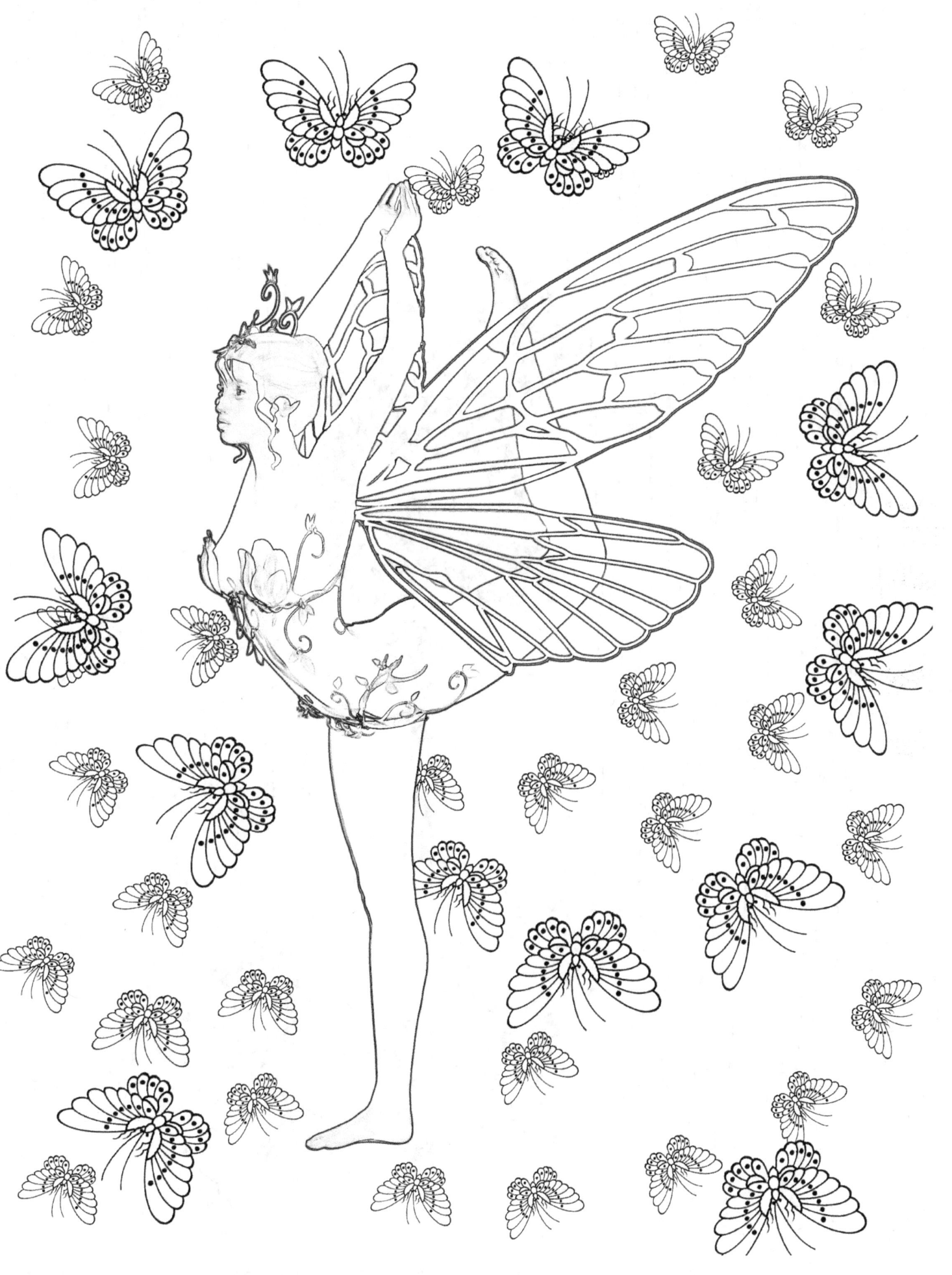

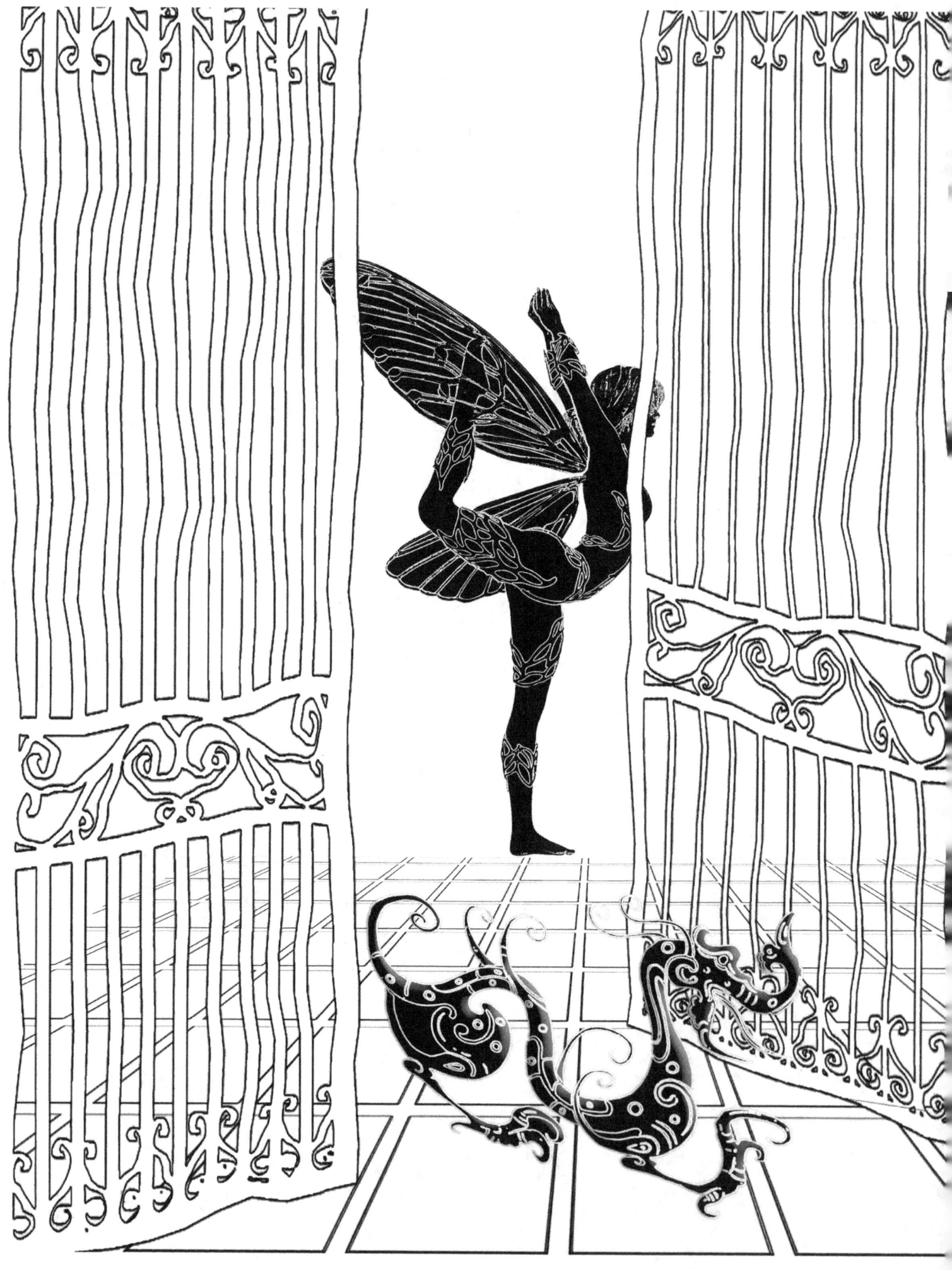

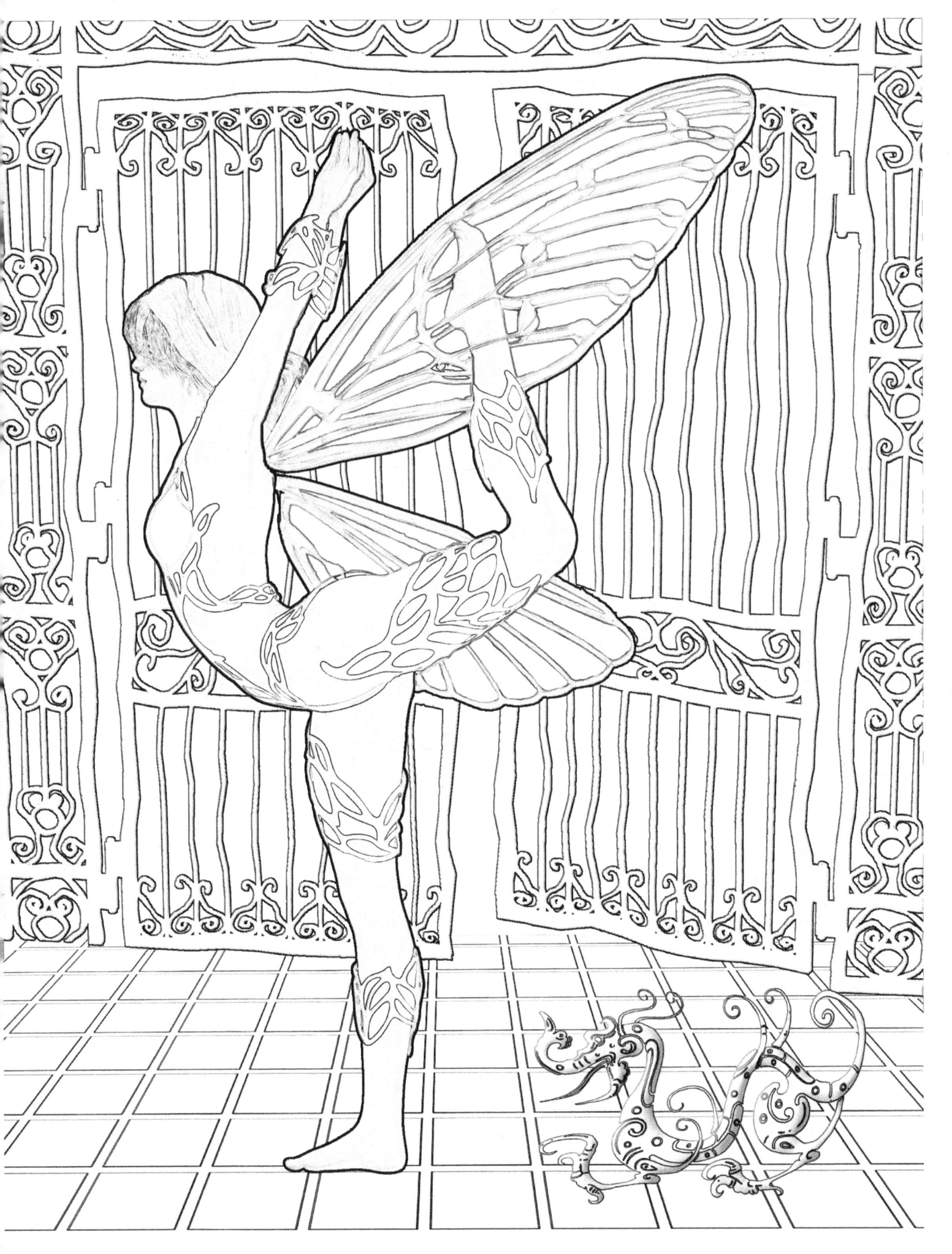

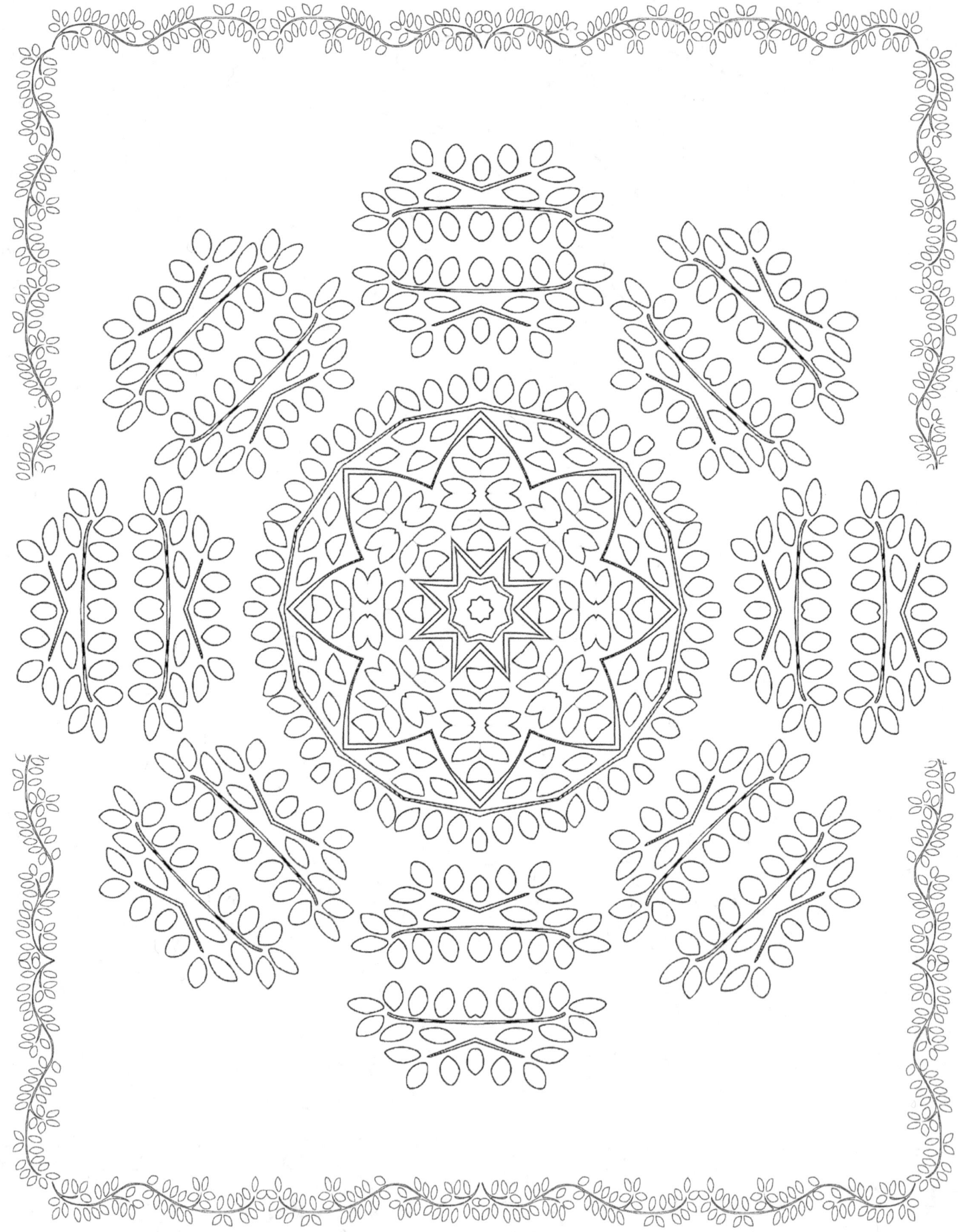

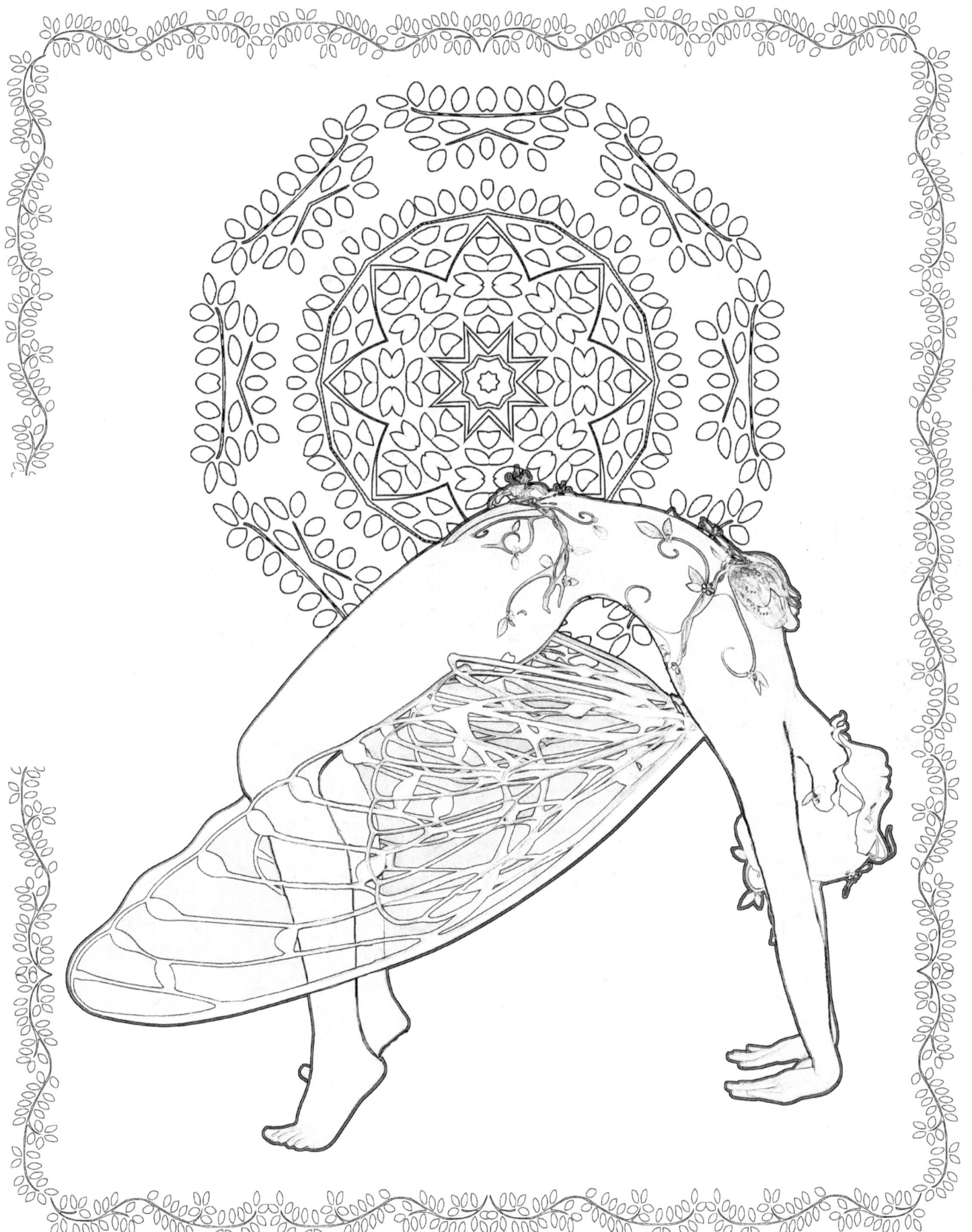

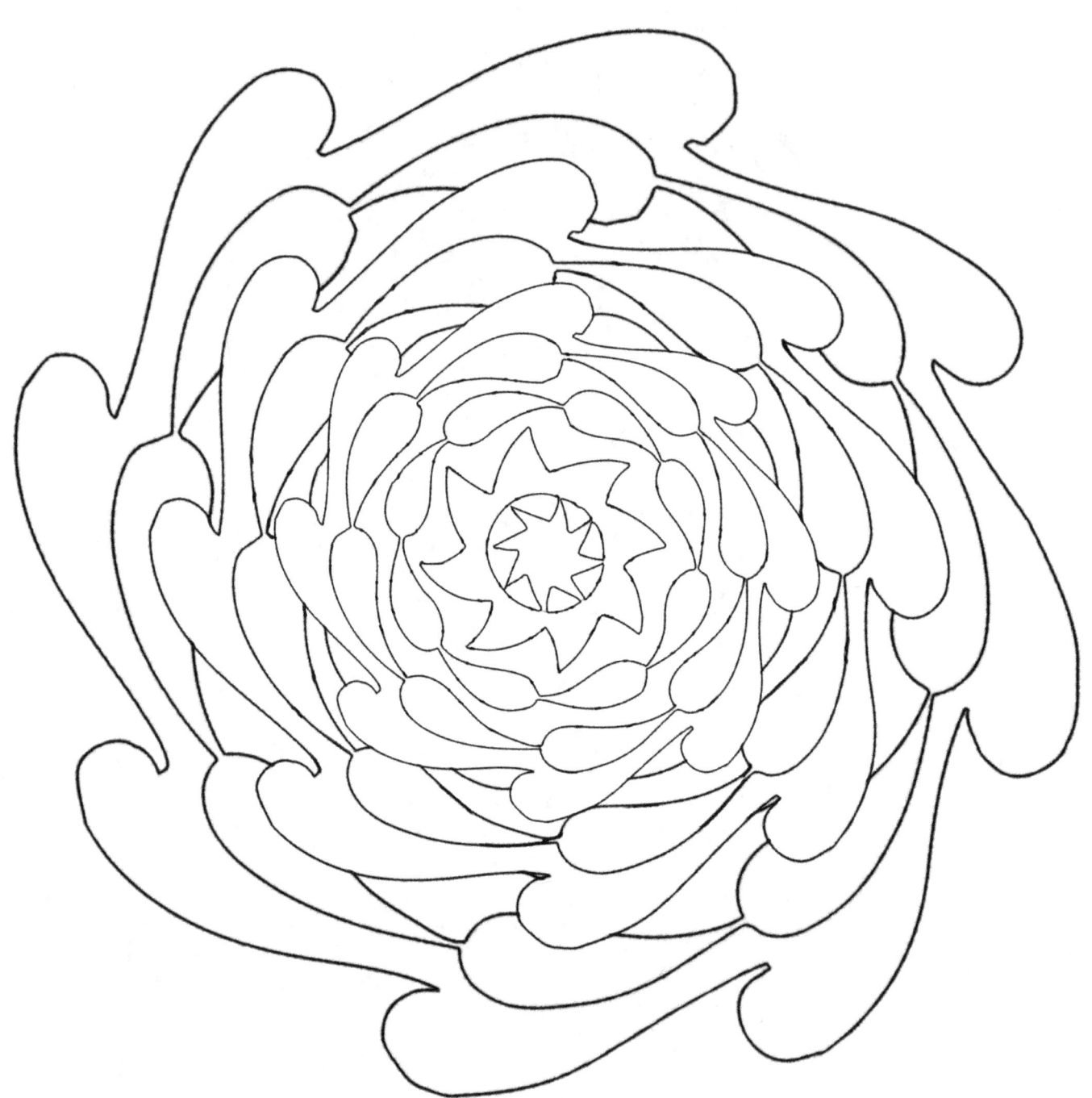

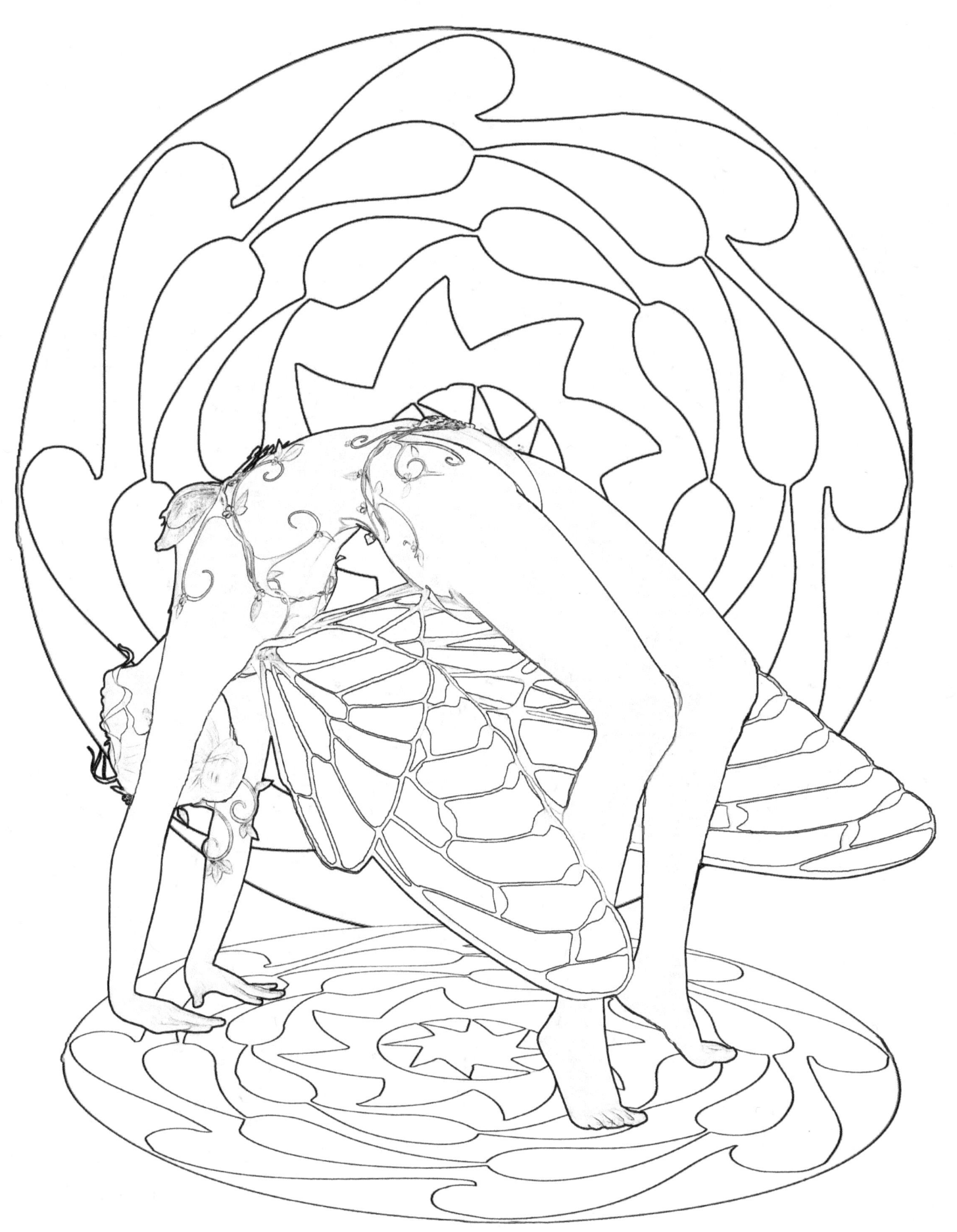

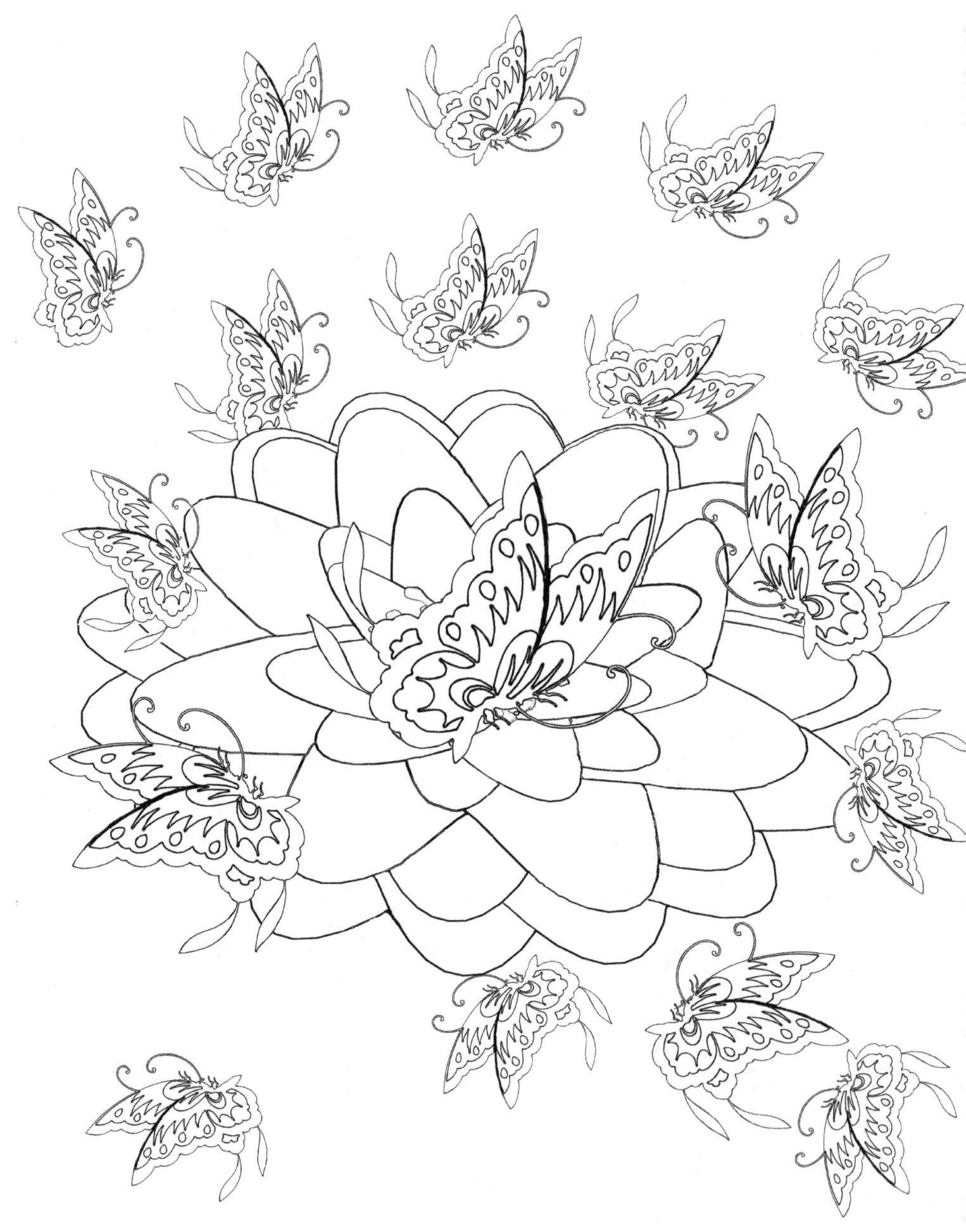

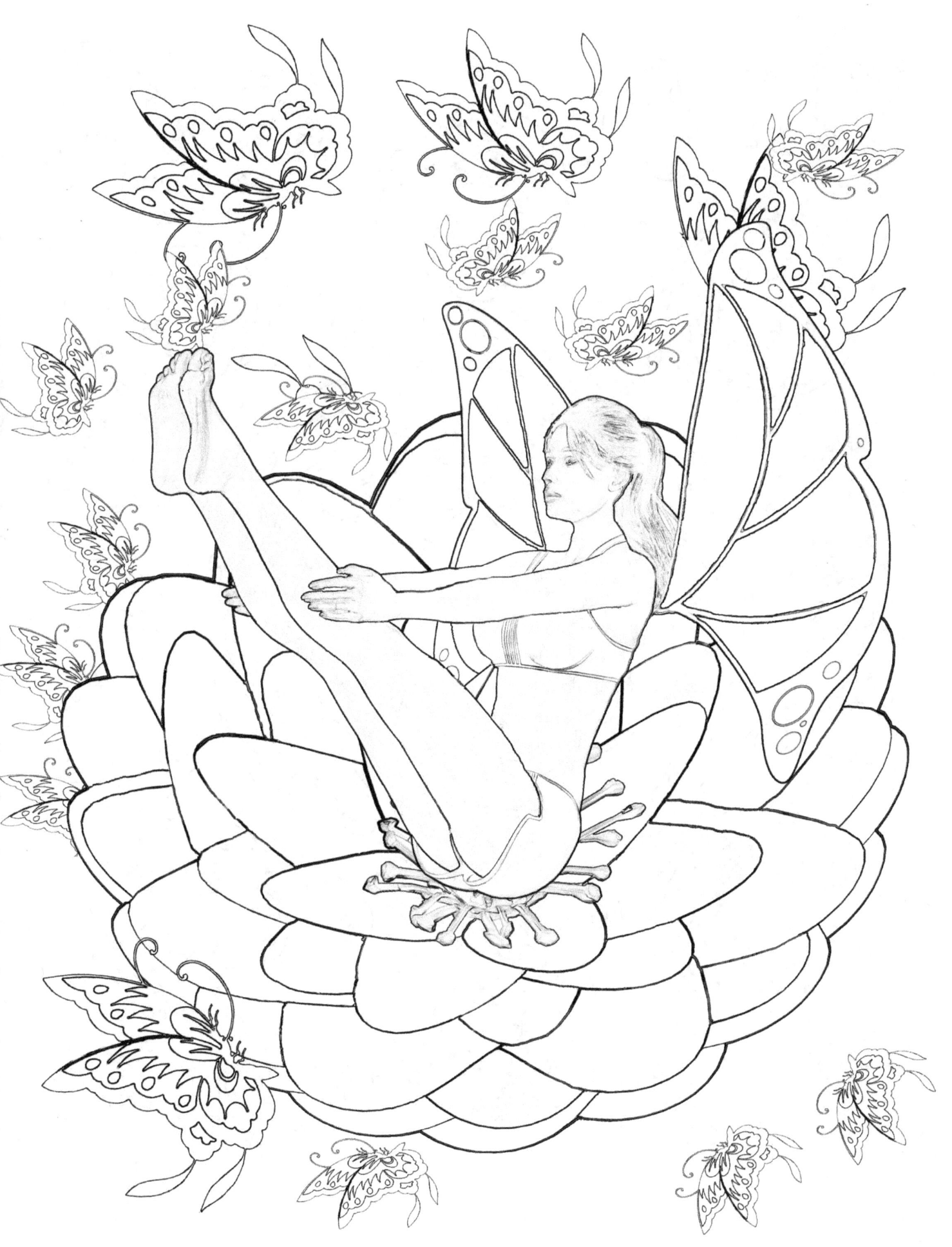

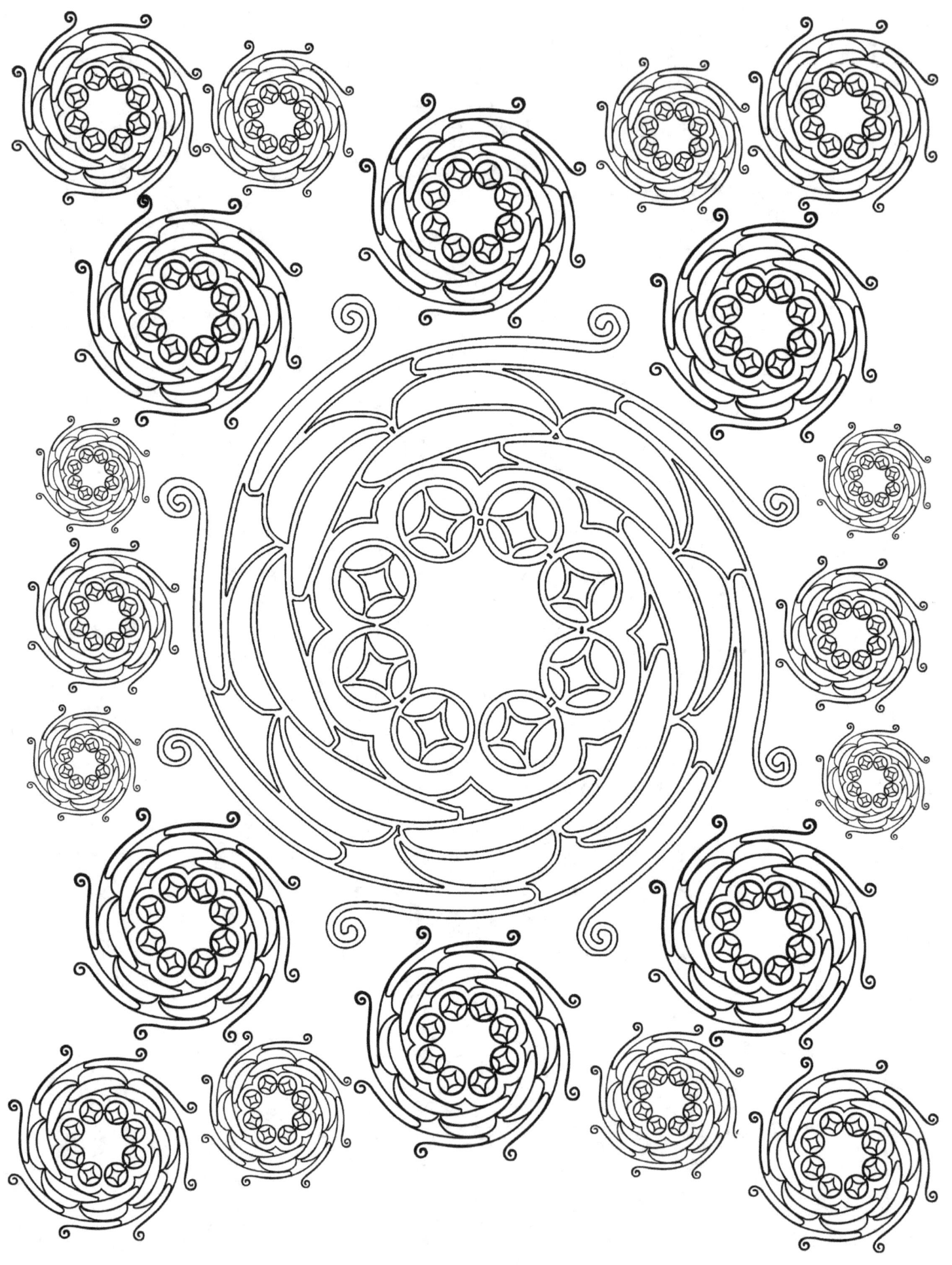

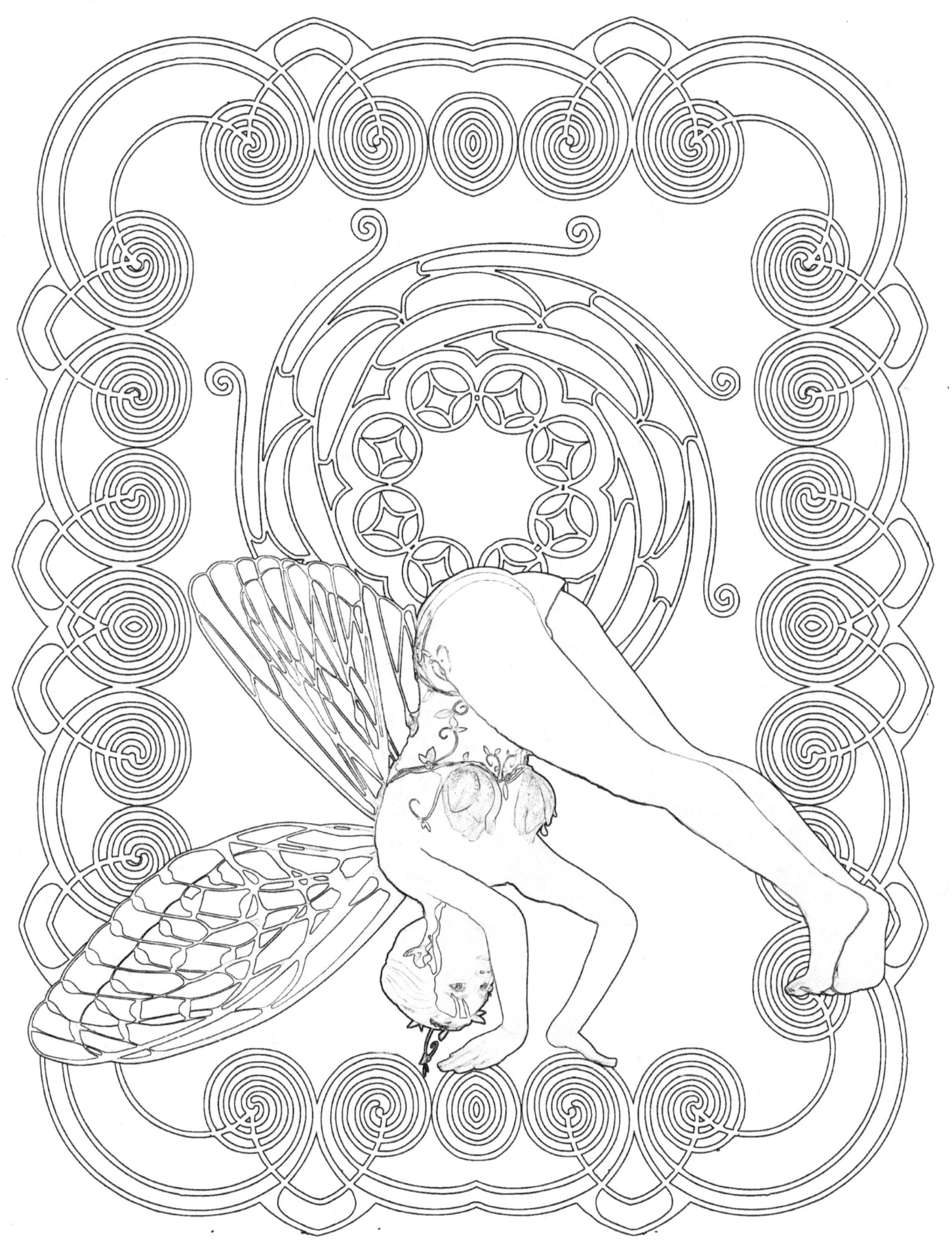

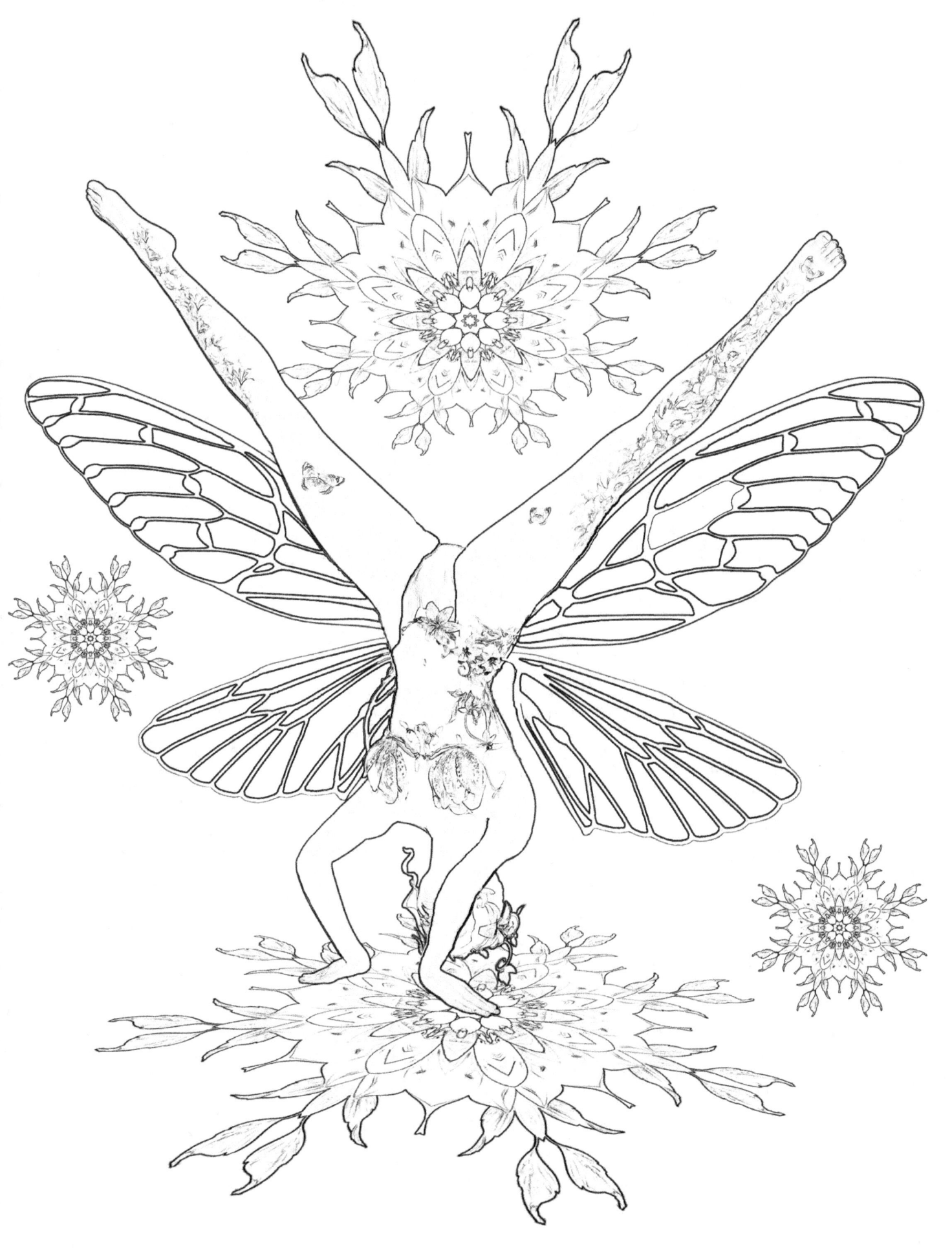

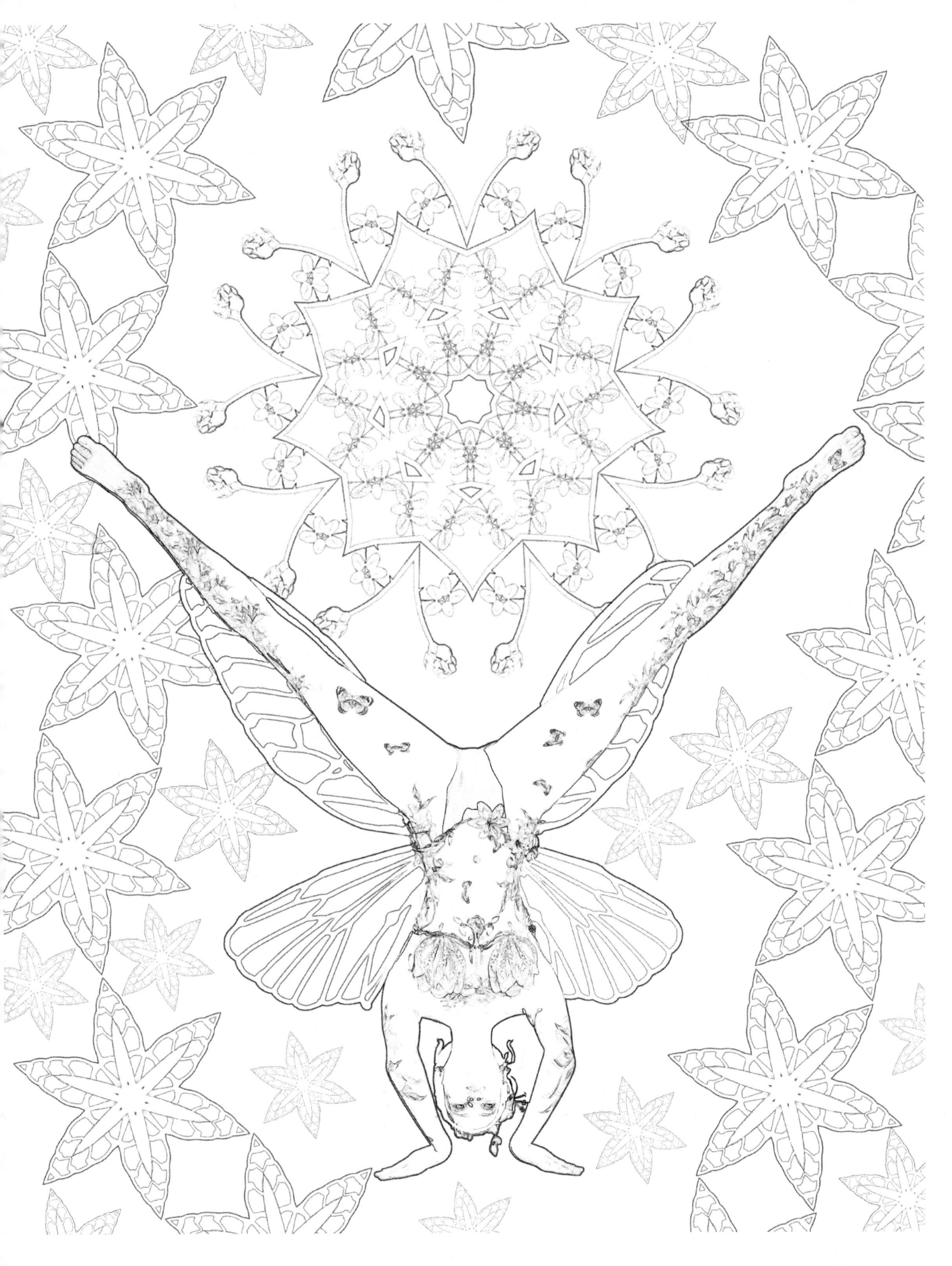

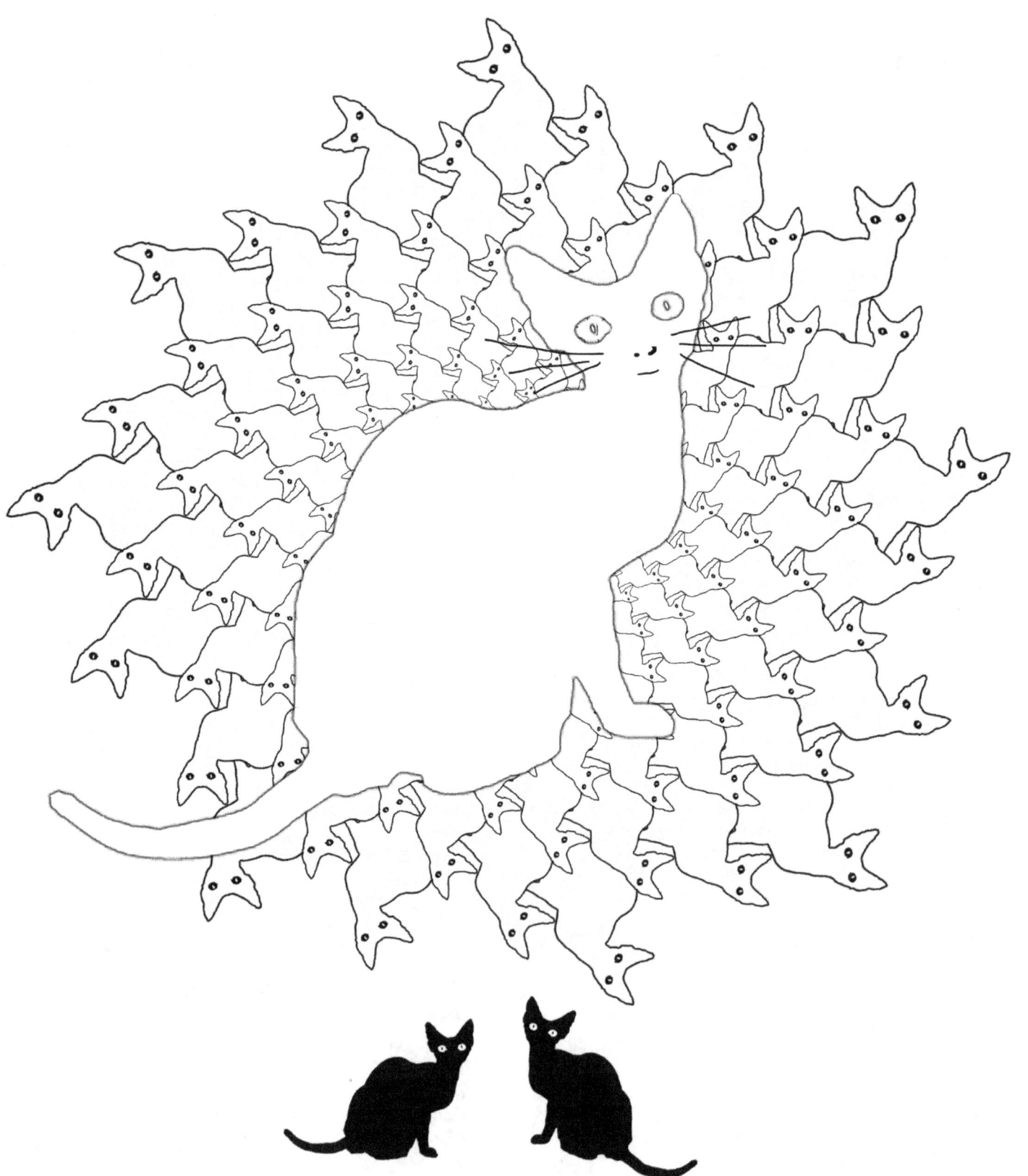

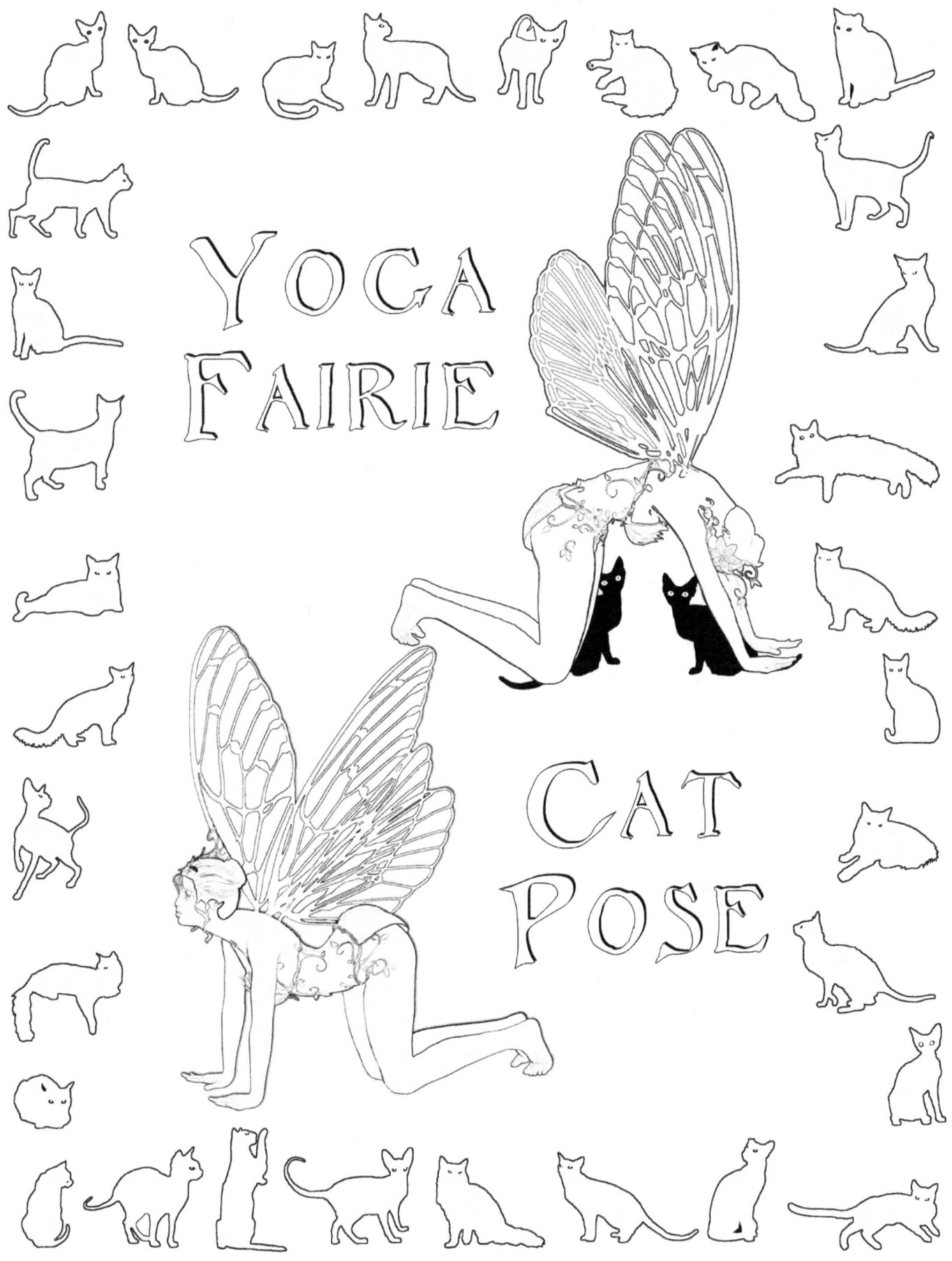

YOGA
FAIRIE

CAT
POSE

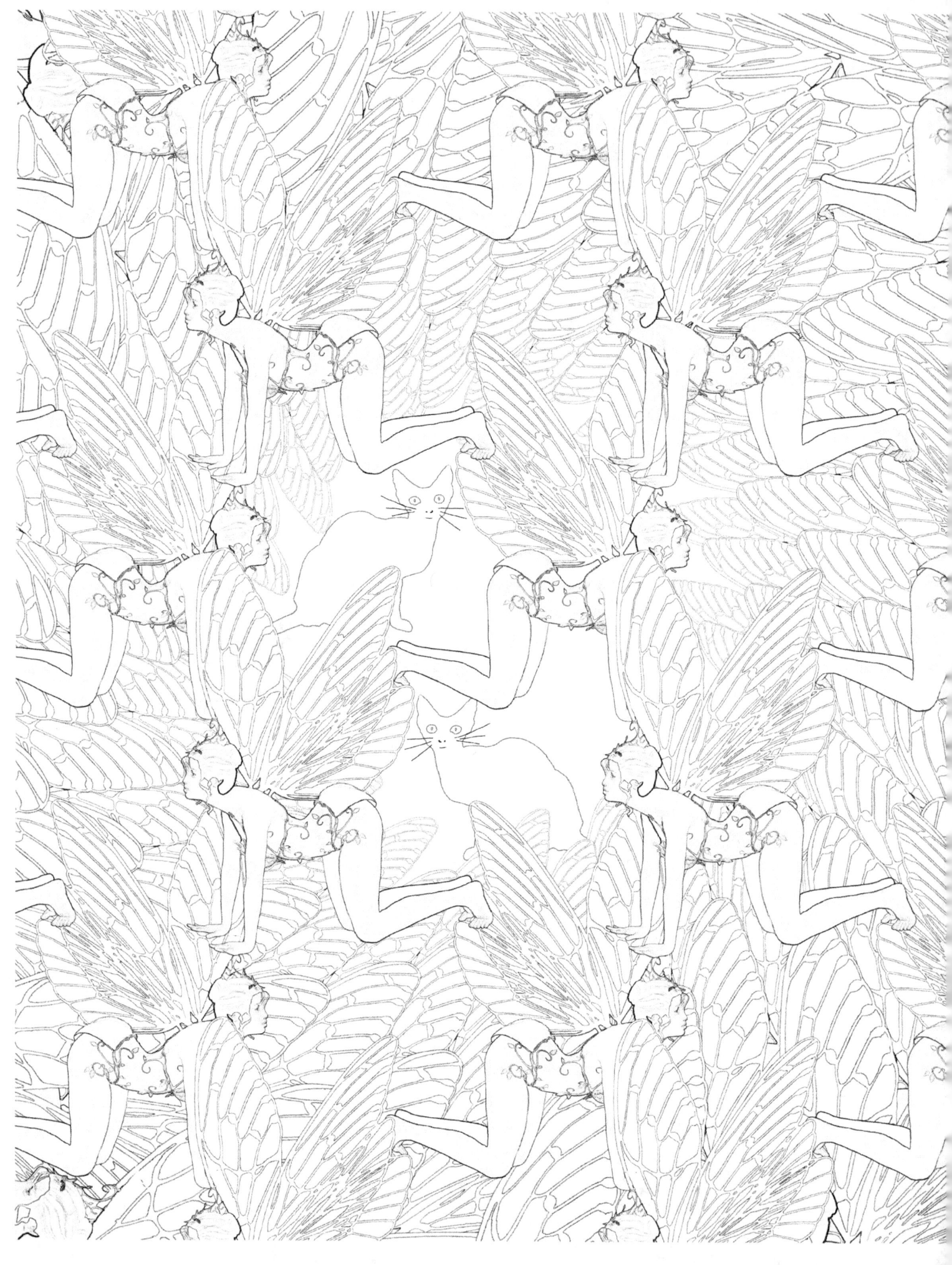

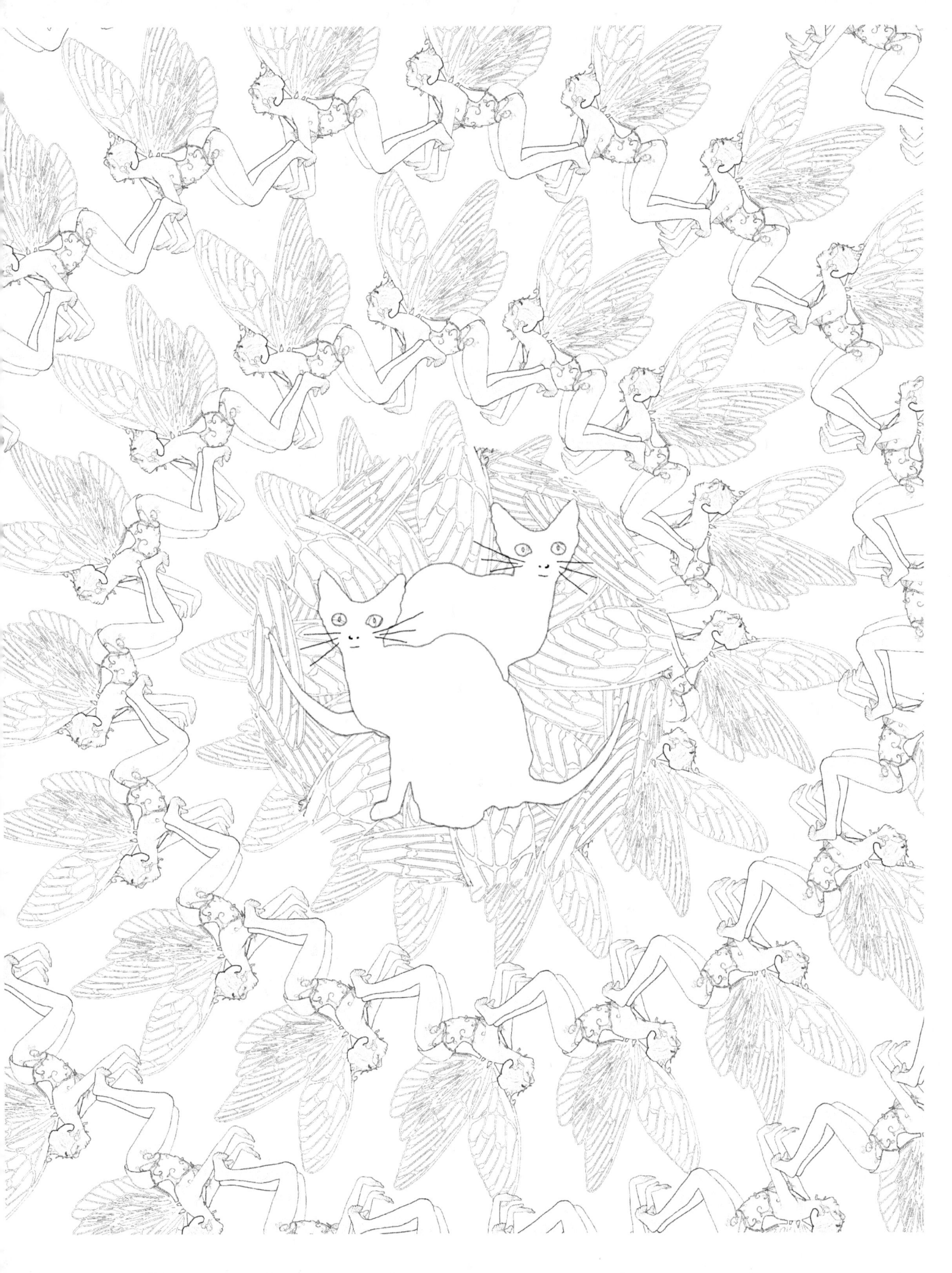

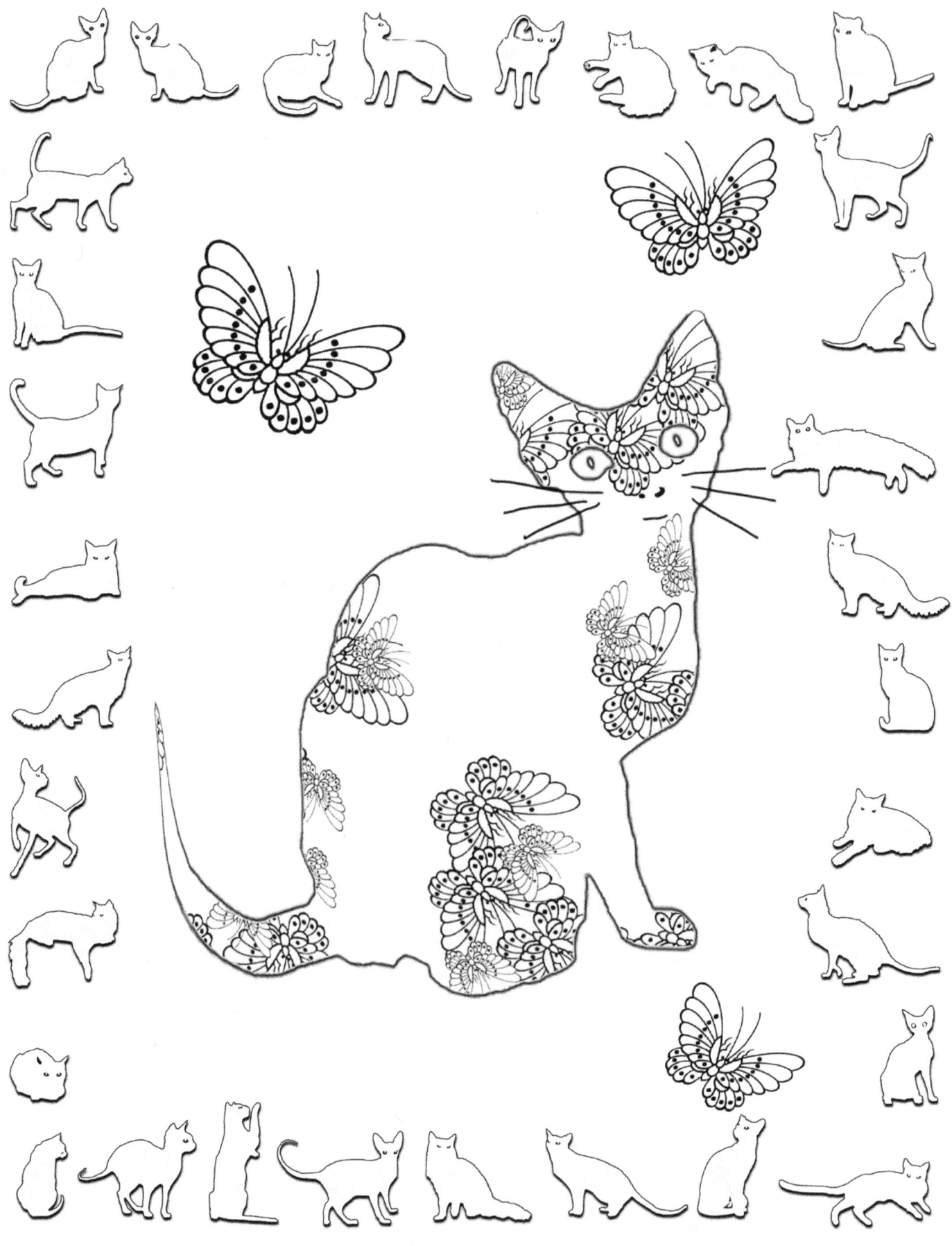

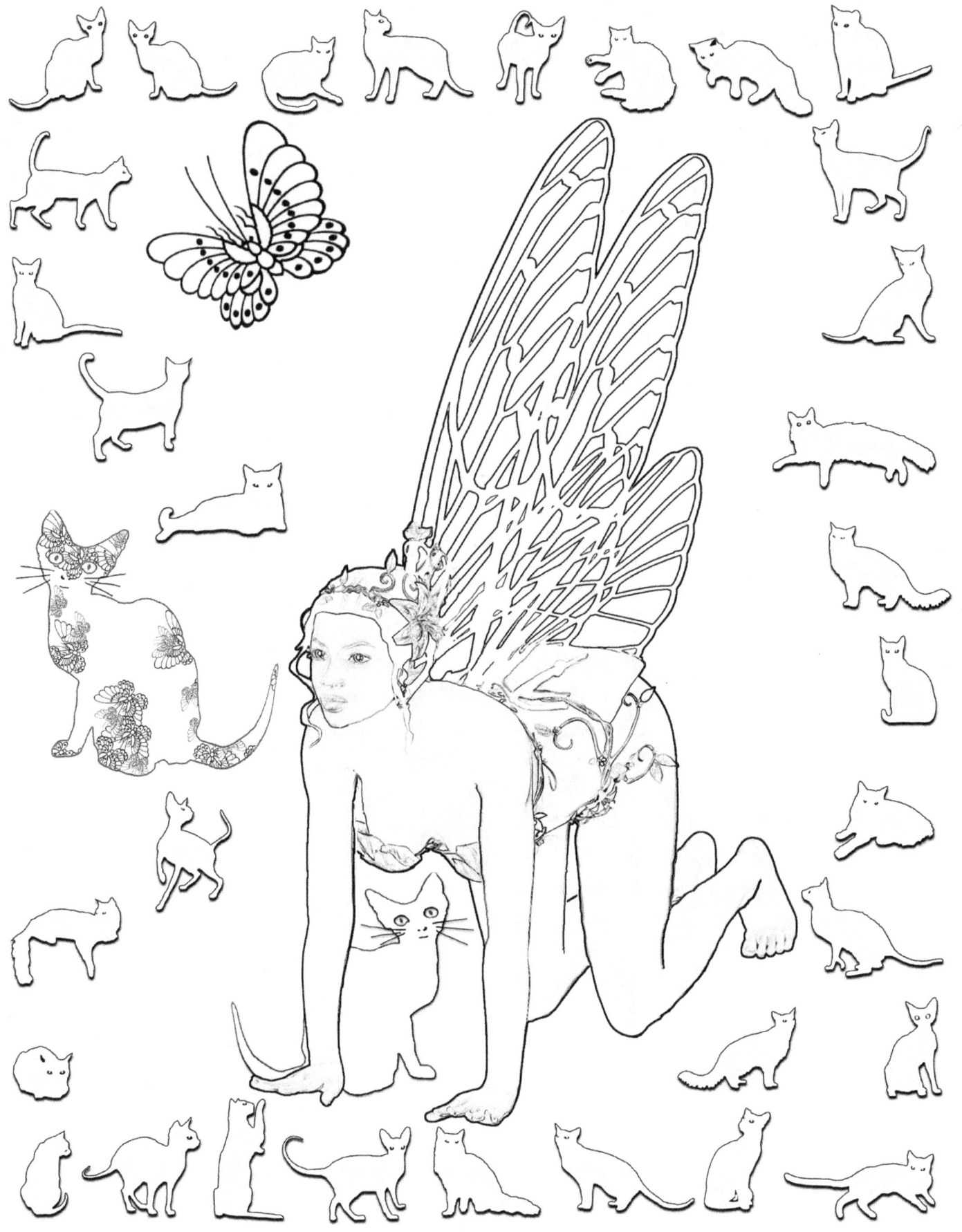

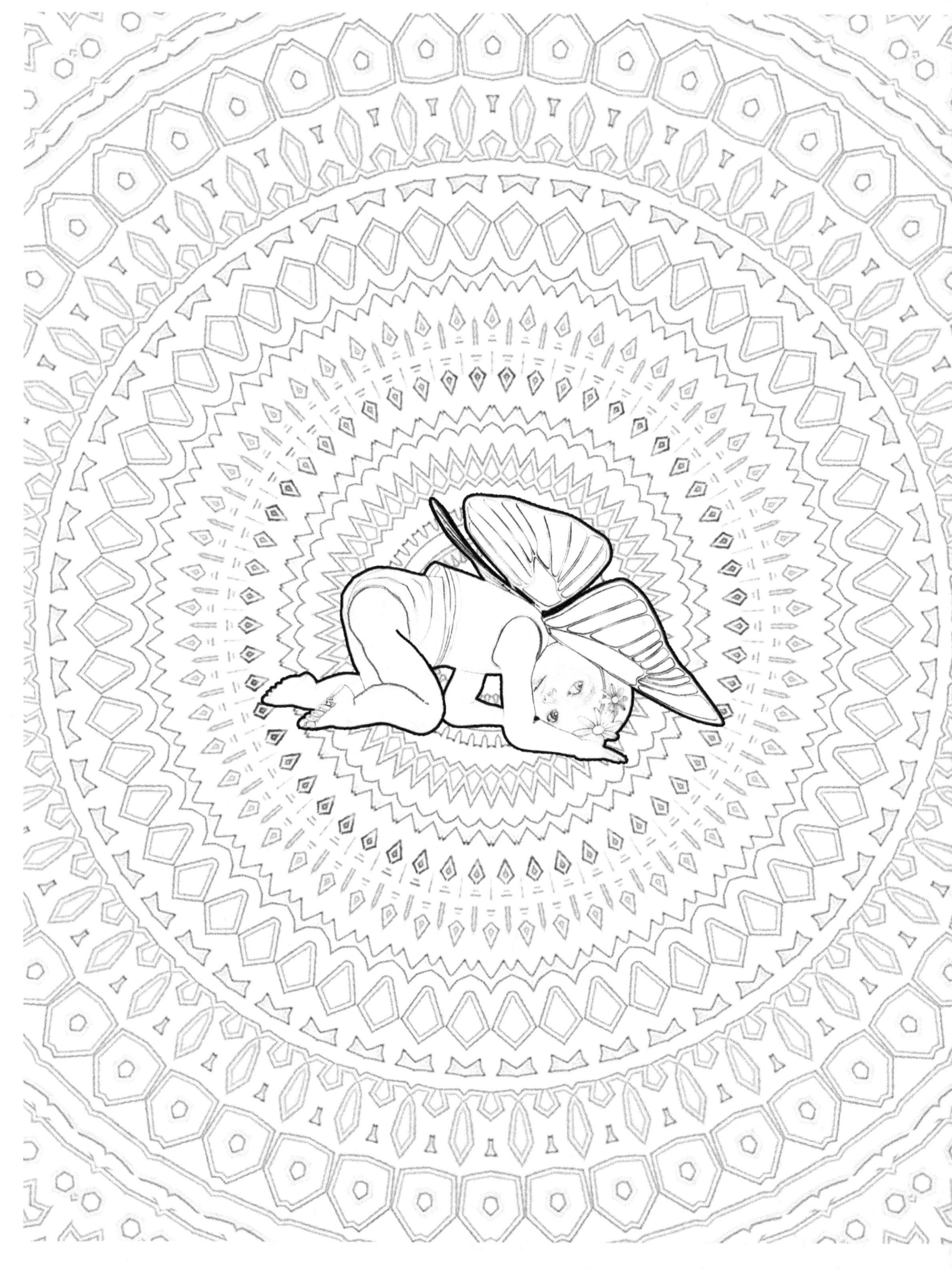

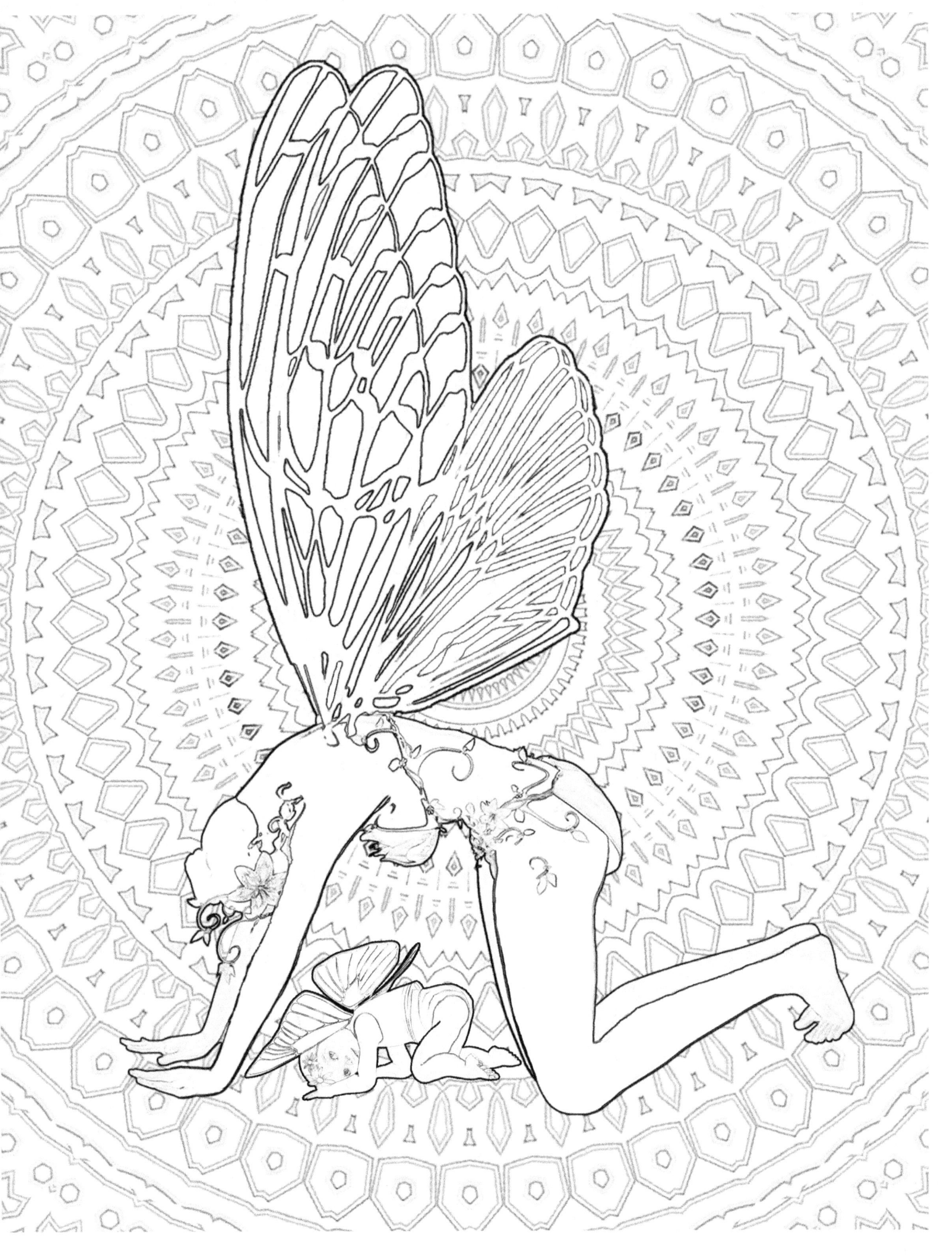

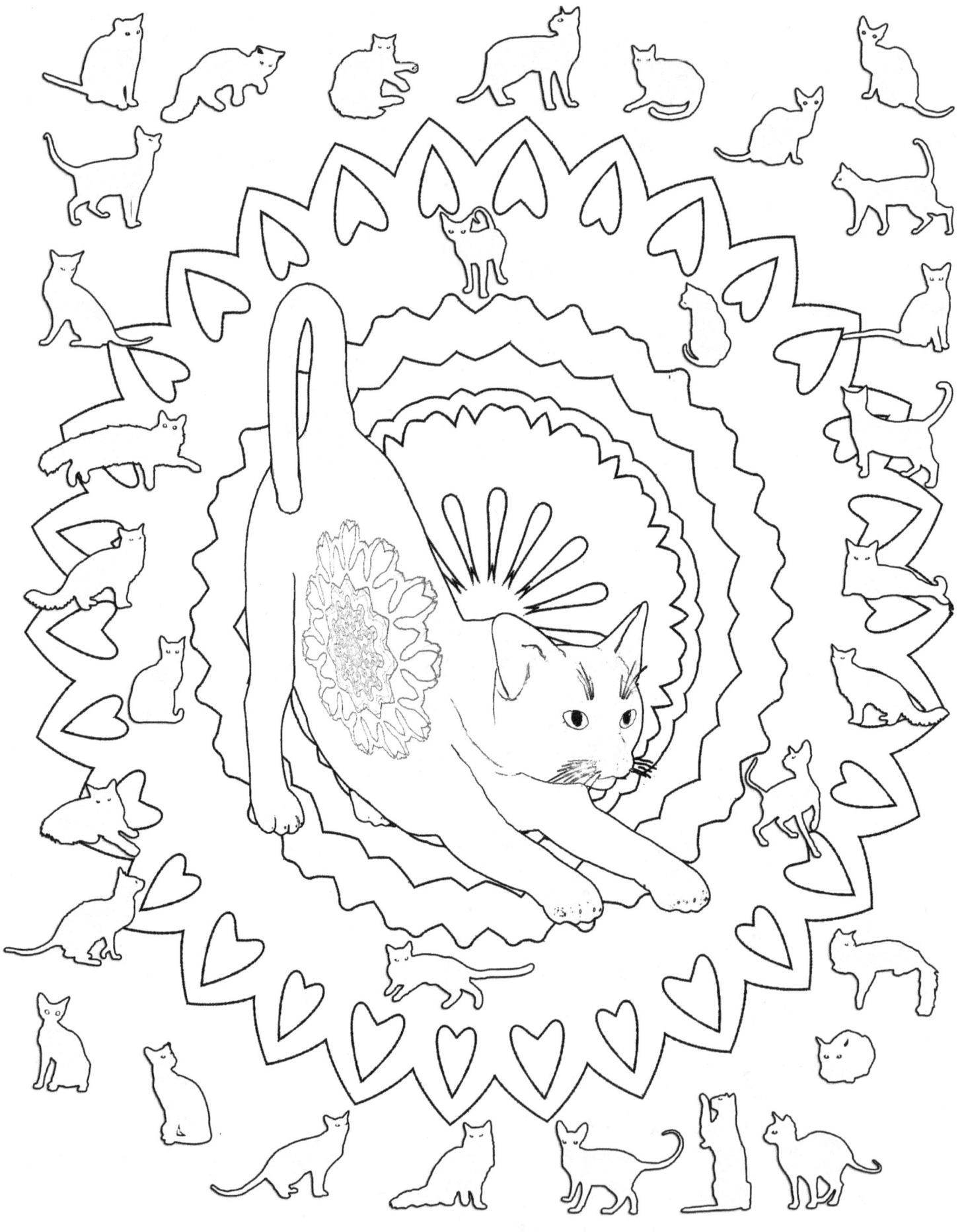

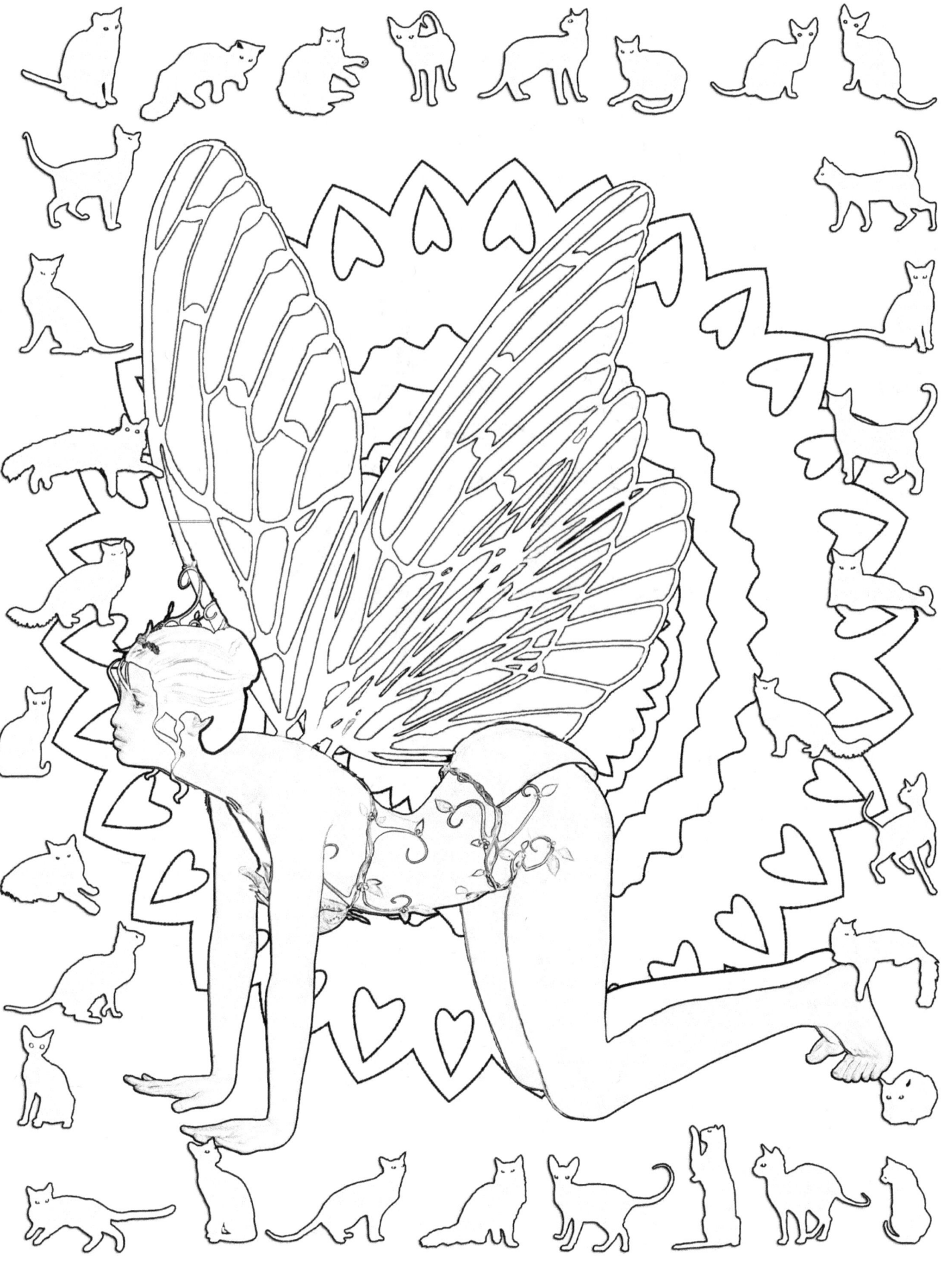

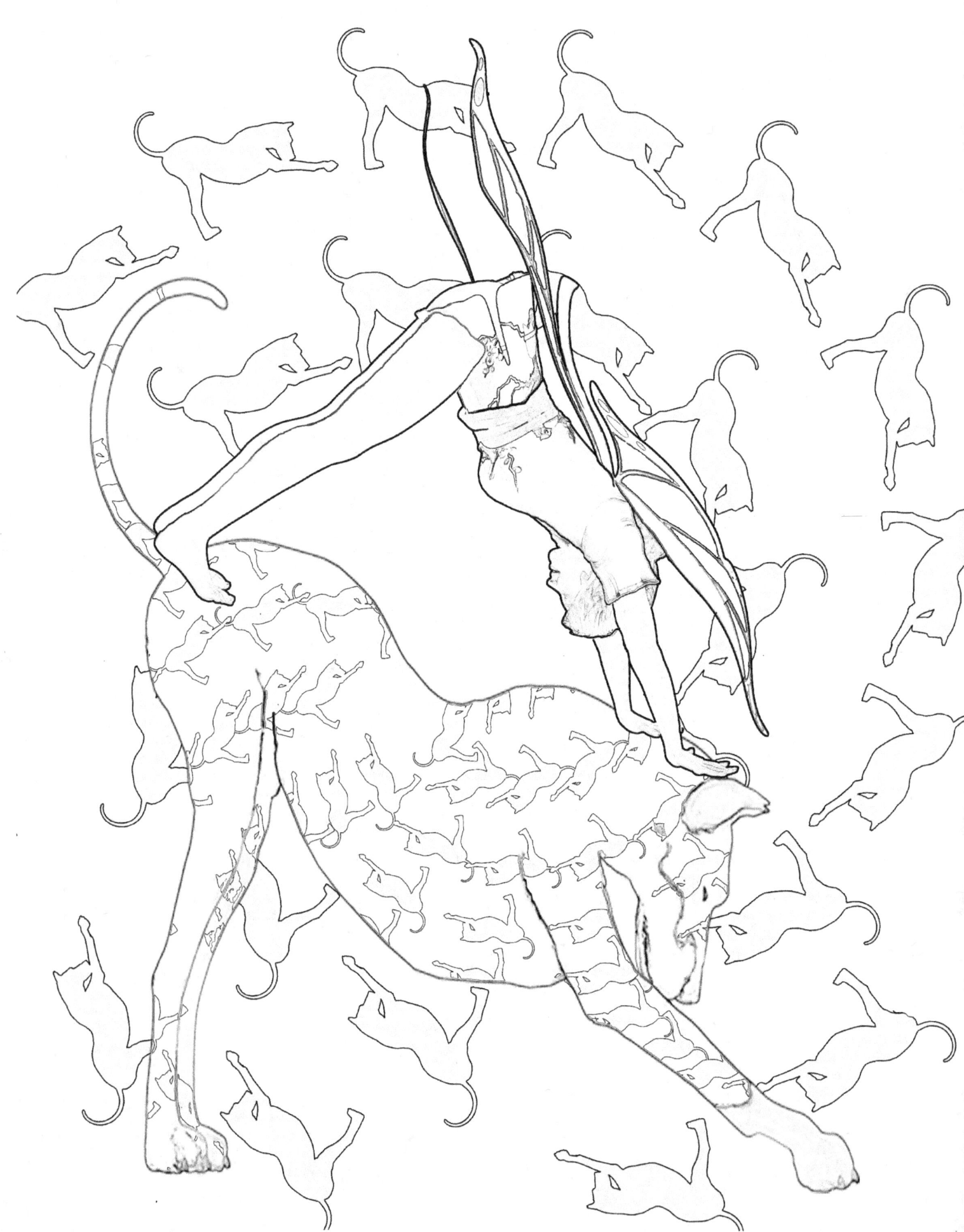

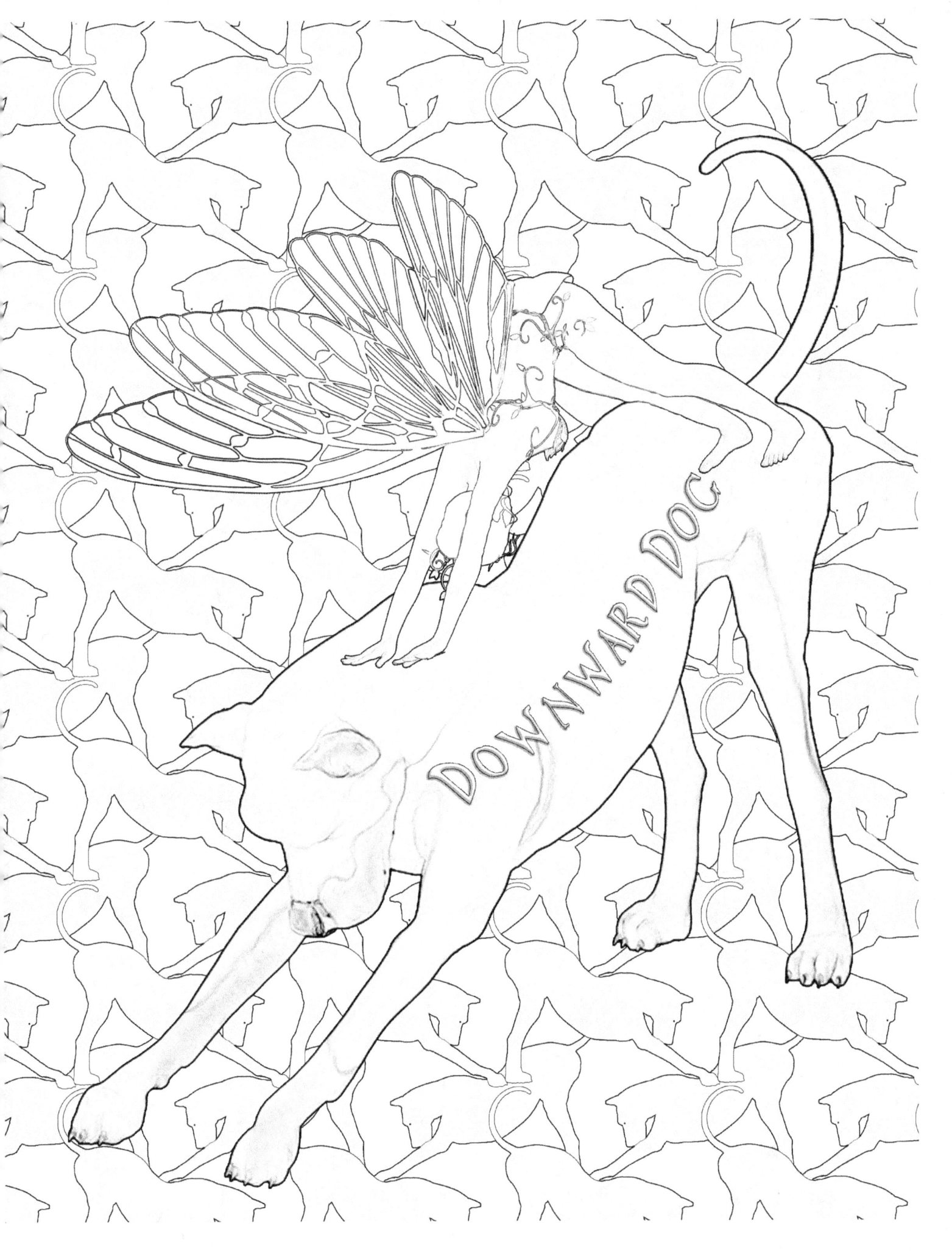

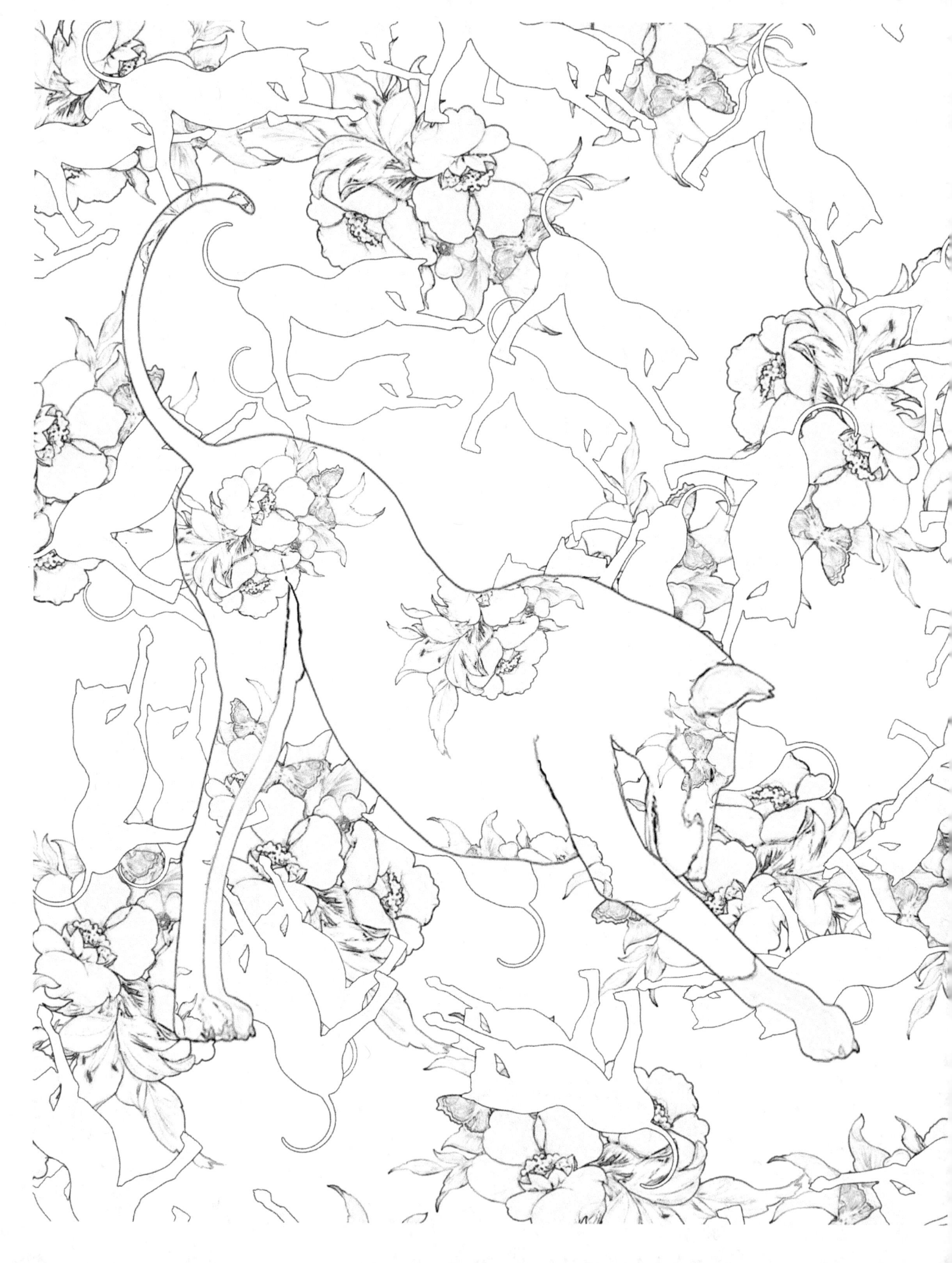

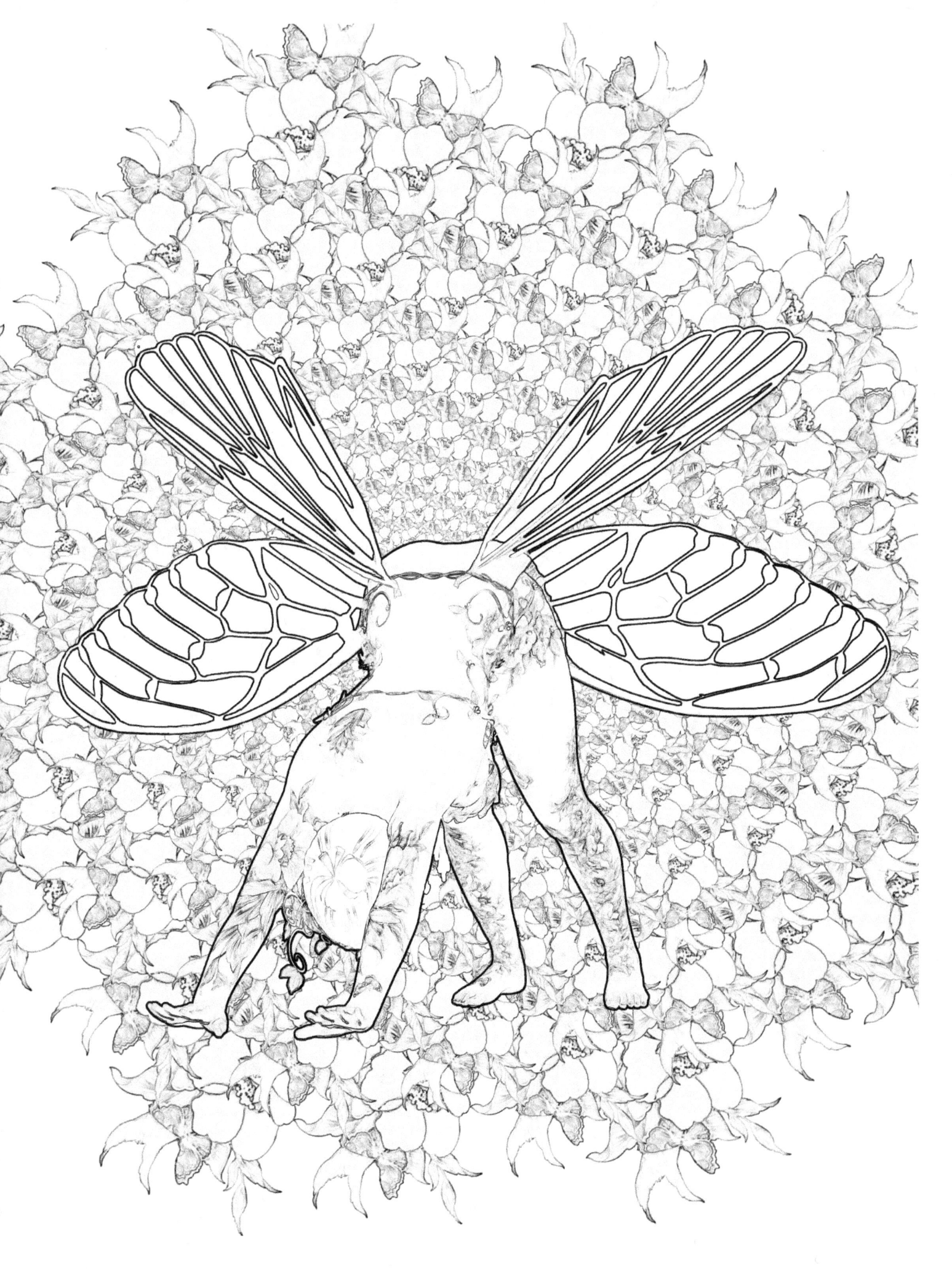

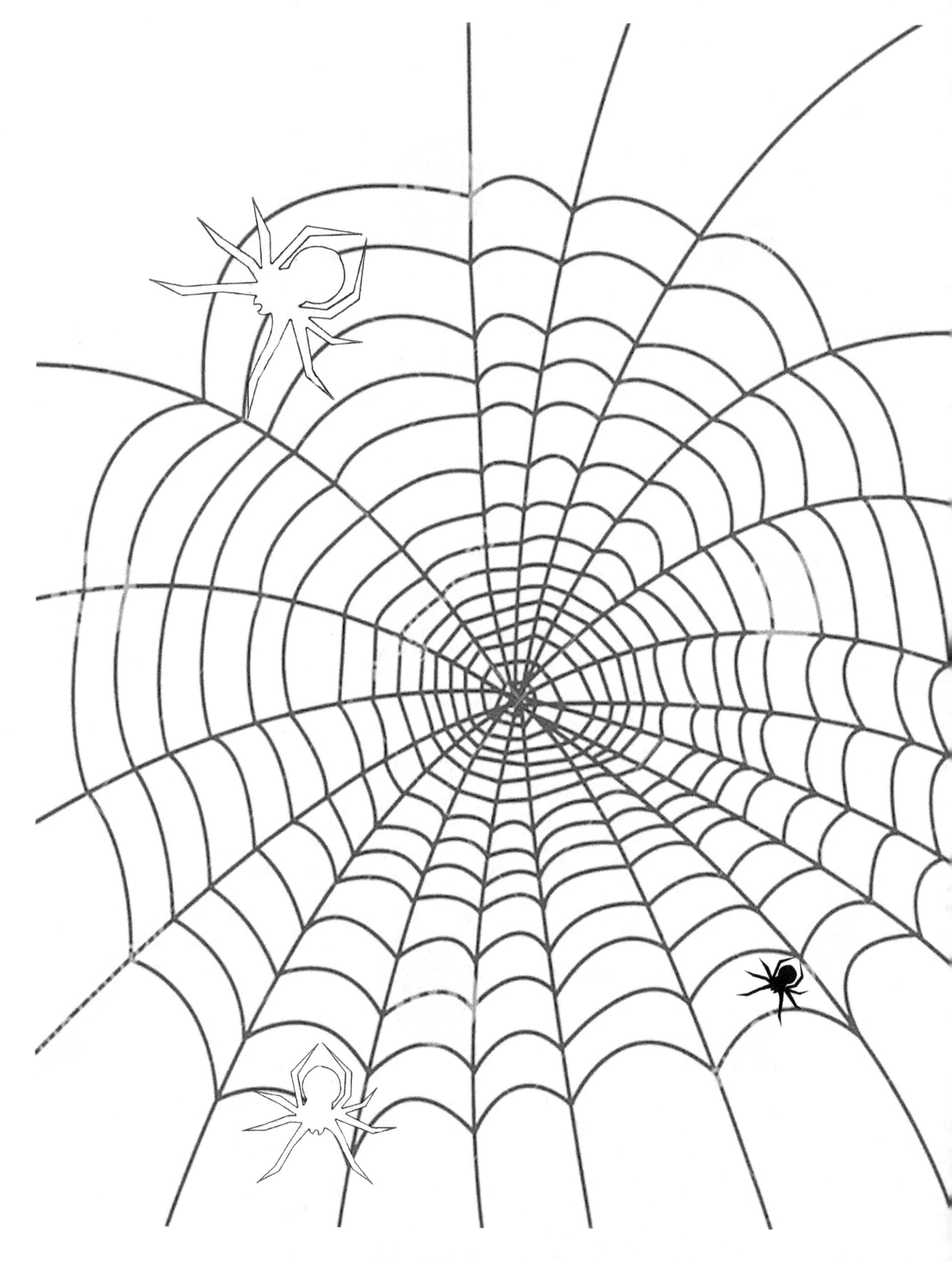

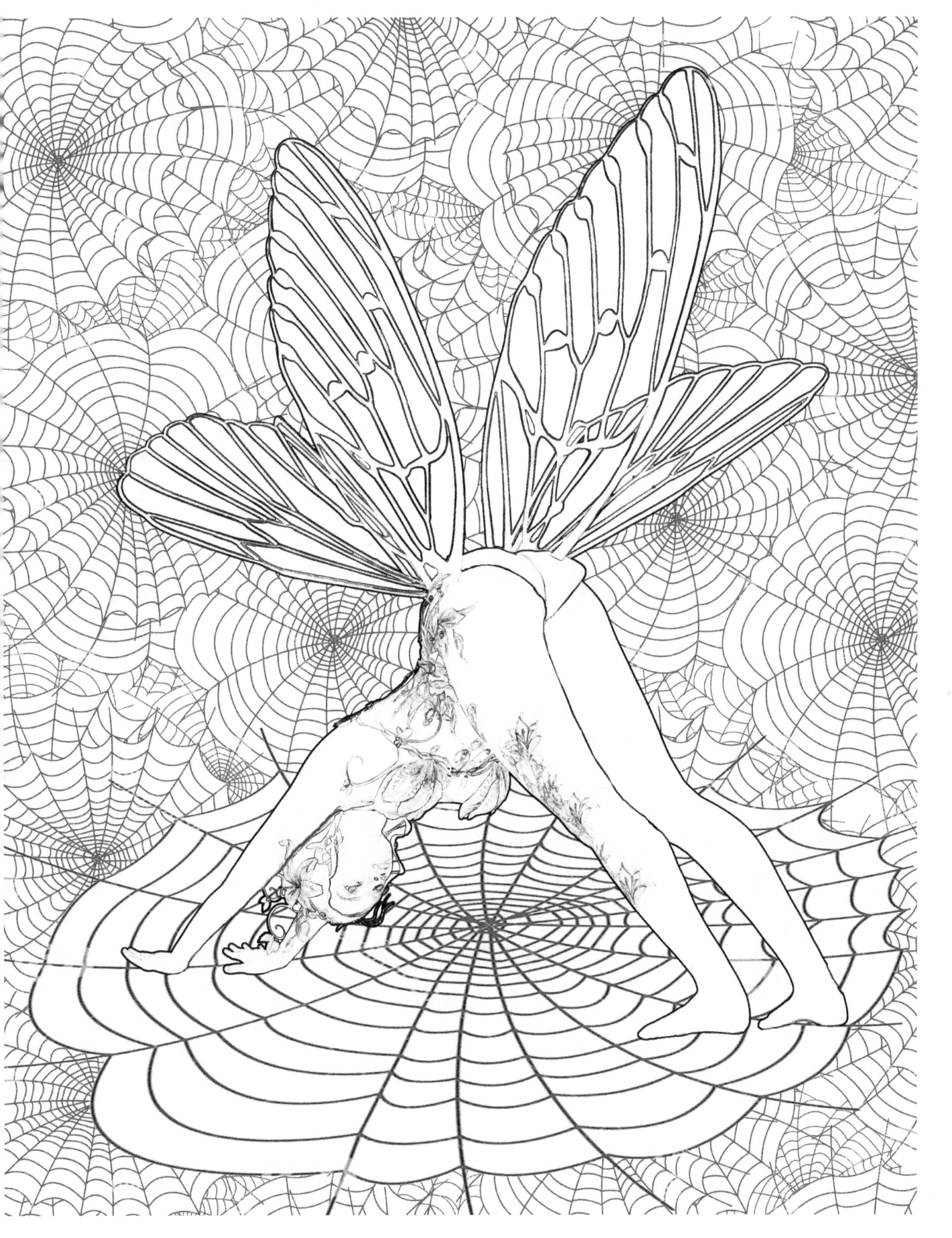

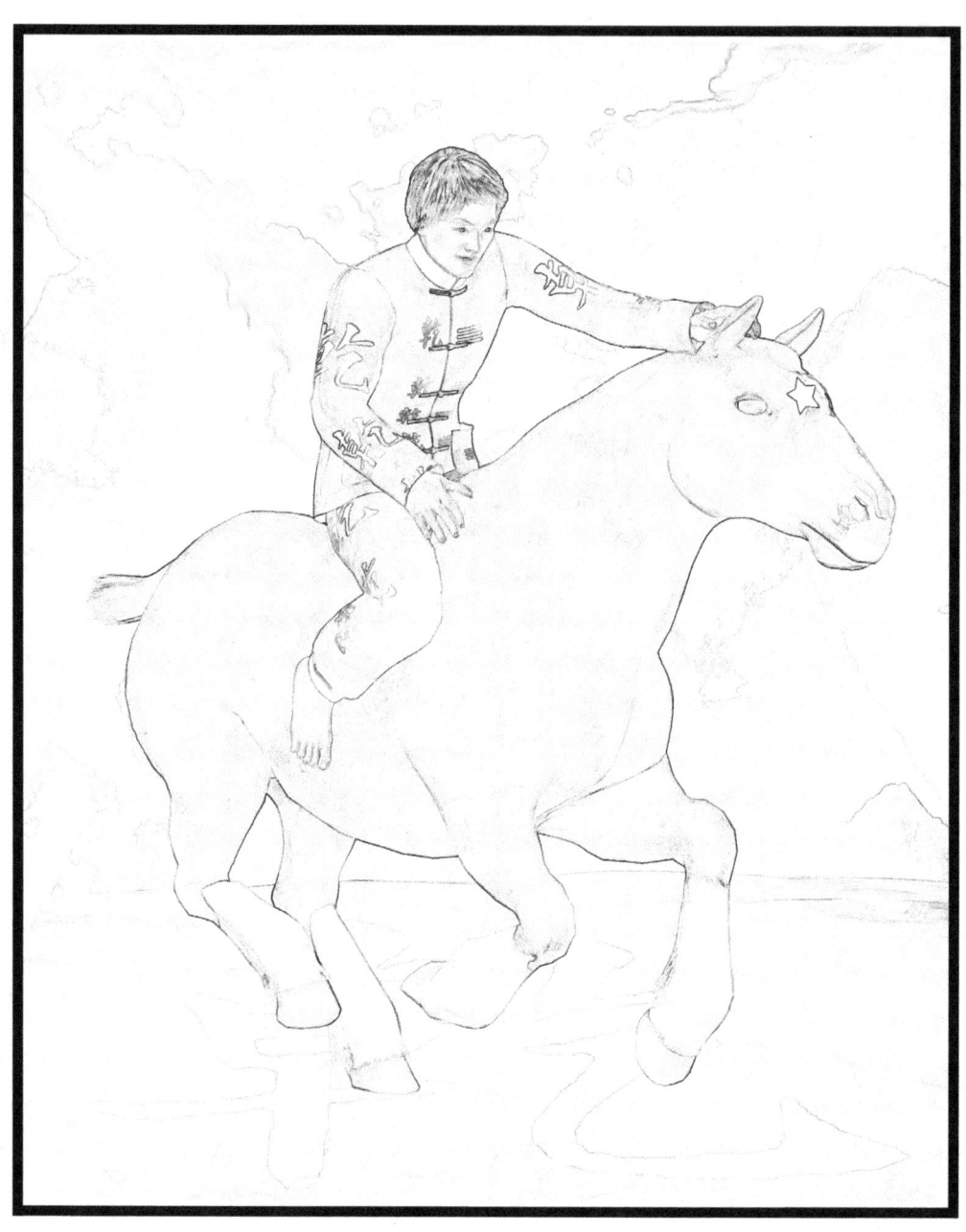

The above image was extracted from the color edition of *I Ching Meditations.*

Adele Aldridge

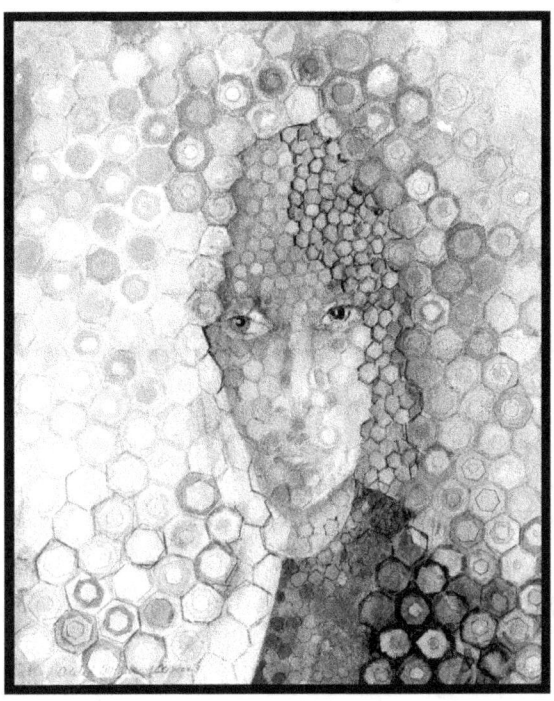

Adele Aldridge has been working with the *I Ching* for 40 years creating images and text for *I Ching Meditations — A Woman's Book of Changes.* She earned a Ph.D. in Art and the Personal Symbolic Process, studying with José Argüelles at the Union Institute University. She has thirty-five years of experience as a fine artist showing her work in galleries in New York, Connecticut and San Francisco. She has worked as a Book Illustrator, Graphic Designer, Web Designer and Instructor in Computer Graphic programs. You can learn more about Adele Aldridge's work with the *I Ching* at: www.ichingmeditations.com.